ARE YOUR PRESCRIPTIONS KILLING YOU?

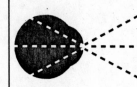

This Large Print Book carries the
Seal of Approval of N.A.V.H.

ARE YOUR PRESCRIPTIONS KILLING YOU?

HOW TO PREVENT DANGEROUS INTERACTIONS, AVOID DEADLY SIDE EFFECTS, AND BE HEALTHIER WITH FEWER DRUGS

ARMON B. NEEL, JR., PHARMD, CGP, AND BILL HOGAN

THORNDIKE PRESS

A part of Gale, Cengage Learning

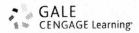
GALE
CENGAGE Learning®

Detroit • New York • San Francisco • New Haven, Conn • Waterville, Maine • London

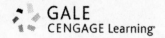

GALE
CENGAGE Learning

Thorndike Press® Large Print Health, Home & Learning.
The text of this Large Print edition is unabridged.
Other aspects of the book may vary from the original edition.
Set in 16 pt. Plantin.

LIBRARY OF CONGRESS CATALOGING-IN-PUBLICATION DATA

Neel, Armon B., author.
   Are your prescriptions killing you? : how to prevent dangerous interactions, avoid deadly side effects, and be healthier with fewer drugs / by Armon B. Neel, Jr., PharmD, CGP, and Bill Hogan. — Large print edition.
   pages cm
   Originally published: New York : Atria Books, 2012.
   ISBN-13: 978-1-4104-5213-9 (hardcover)
   ISBN-10: 1-4104-5213-1 (hardcover) 1. Drugs—Popular works. 2. Drug interactions—Popular works. 3. Drugs—Side effects—Popular works. 4. Large type books. I. Hogan, Bill, 1953 June 23– II. Title.
   RM302.5.N44 2012b
   615.7'045—dc23   2012025891

Published in 2012 by arrangement with Atria Books, a division of Simon & Schuster, Inc.

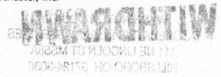

Printed in Mexico
2 3 4 5 6 7 16 15 14 13 12

To James R. Westbury Sr., a very dear friend who always believed in my vision and, most comforting of all, always believed in me.

— A.N.

To my family and to Armon, with the hope that through this book, his courage and wisdom can touch many more lives.

— B.H.

CONTENTS

PROLOGUE:
THE PHARMACIST WHO
SAYS NO TO DRUGS
BY BILL HOGAN

Ruby Gifford has come to see Armon Neel Jr. out of fear and perhaps even desperation. Gifford, eighty-six, hasn't been feeling well lately, and the long list of symptoms that have prompted her to travel to Neel's office in Griffin, Georgia, on a sunny day in the summer of 2004 might well mark her as a hypochondriac in the eyes of many doctors. Her problems run from dizzy spells and falls to osteoarthritis and back pain, and then from high blood pressure and low pulse rates to anxiety and depression. Then there are the skin rashes, hives, and other allergic symptoms that seem to have come out of nowhere.

Gifford's sixty-year-old daughter has brought her to the Wednesday morning appointment, and the two wait anxiously in Neel's conference room, where he meets with patients. Neel, however, isn't a doctor. He's a pharmacist whose specialty is determining whether people are taking the right medications — and in the right doses — for what ails them. Neel hasn't worked behind a prescription counter since the late 1970s, when he gave up dispensing drugs for a career that would put him on a collision course, often, with the doctors who prescribe them.

After introducing himself to the two women, Neel breaks the ice with some small talk about his seven-year-old grandson's aptitude with computers. His down-home Georgia drawl and courtly manner clearly put his visitors at ease. He makes the point that old age is just old age — nothing more, nothing less — by telling the story of a 102-year-old patient in a nursing home who could break out of her severe dementia to play a concert-quality rendition of Debussy's "Clair de Lune" on the piano. "You never get too old to learn," Neel says.

"If I could find out what's causing all these allergies," Gifford tells him, "I wouldn't mind living that long."

Neel asks to see the blood pressure log she's been keeping for the past couple of weeks at his request ("You did a good job," he tells her), along with all the medications she's been taking. Gifford reaches down, pulls out a freezer-size Ziploc bag that's bulging with prescription drugs, and places it on the table. Then out comes another Ziploc bag full of the over-the-counter medications.

"My doctor doesn't know what to do with me," Gifford says. "I never had any allergies like this."

Neel quizzes Gifford about the prescription drugs one by one. "What about that?" he asks. "How did that one do?"

He asks Gifford about Ultracet, a pain medication that she's taking that's part tramadol, part acetaminophen. "I never have headaches," she says. "My aches are all from falls."

"Tell me about the falls," Neel says. "Tell me how long it was after taking this pill that it happened."

Neel gently guides Gifford through the entire list. He explains that Aldactone, the blood pressure medication she's been taking, isn't the drug of choice in her case and may, in fact, be responsible for some of her other health problems. (It can cause dizziness, confusion, and skin rashes, among other adverse effects.) As he looks through Gifford's records, he sees that her doctor, in an attempt to control her hypertension, has tried four different ACE inhibitors, two beta-blockers, and two alpha-blockers.

13

Nothing has worked, and Gifford has experienced allergic reactions to all of them. Neel seems stupefied. "There wasn't a need to go to the second one after the first one did you harm," he says. "They're in the same family. You need a calcium channel blocker instead."

Next, Neel zeroes in on Mobic, the NSAID (nonsteroidal anti-inflammatory drug) that Gifford's doctor has prescribed for her osteoarthritis. "There are certain drugs you just don't give old people," he explains, and NSAIDs are among them. It turns out that her doctor has ordered yet another NSAID, in the form of Voltaren ophthalmic drops. "There's a newer product that's better than this," Neel says.

Gifford seems relieved but at the same time disturbed. "I don't want to go back to this doctor," she says. "She never checked anything before she gave it to me. She has a nice bedside manner, but I don't want to go back to her."

Neel promises to put everything in a written report by the end of the week. "Some of these things," he says, pointing to all the medications spread out on the table, "we might just chuck in the trash can."

Neel will hit the road later in the day to

make his way to two nursing homes in rural Georgia, where he will review the charts of dozens of residents and carry on his long-running crusade against the overmedication of geriatric patients in long-term care facilities. Neel does this two or three days a week, nearly every week, and has been doing it virtually nonstop since 1977, when he decided to focus entirely on clinical consulting. He's one of a relatively small number of consultant pharmacists nationwide who specialize in identifying, resolving, and preventing medication-related problems that affect, and afflict, older people.

At around six o'clock Neel steps outside his office in downtown Griffin, packs a few things in the tiny trunk of his 1999 Mazda Miata, drops his six-foot-three frame into the driver's seat, and slips on his sunglasses. Neel, sixty-six, used to cruise the state in a late-model Cadillac, but now the sleek little Miata — a rare "10th Anniversary" model with an eye-catching sapphire-blue paint job — is both a point of pride for Neel and the thing that makes his hours on the road bearable, if not pleasurable. While driving through the Georgia countryside, he sips Diet Dr Pepper nonstop, listens to the kind of music no one of his generation has been known to like (techno, mostly, and other electronic dance music), and thinks about the work that is also his life.

In his own profession, Neel is a rebel with a cause: namely, advancing the idea that pharmacists are to serve and protect the people who take the medications they dispense. ("When I get paid," he says, "I get paid by the patient, not the doc.") The way he sees it, pharmacists are often the patient's last line of defense in a nation of physicians who, more often than not, don't know much about the drugs they are prescribing.

The renegade streak goes way back. In 1963, for instance, just two years out of pharmacy school, Neel opened an apothecary shop in Griffin that featured a carpeted reception room (just like a doctor's office) and a separate consultation room. He also set up prenatal and postnatal counseling programs, as well as hypertension and diabetes care clinics. Neel thought the new approach would earn praise; instead it drew ridicule from many of his peers. From 1966 to 1977, Neel was hauled before the state pharmacy board six times simply for counseling patients on the proper use of the medications they'd been prescribed. (The pharmacy board never took any action against Neel, and, finally, in 1990

16

Georgia law was changed to allow pharmacists in the state to offer such basic advice.)

In the late 1960s, Neel, at the request of a friend, started doing some clinical consulting in nursing homes, and what he saw both shocked and transformed him. "Here was a brand-new population of people, and nobody had any earthly idea how to take care of them," he recalls. "Back then you'd see Mellaril [the brand name for thioridazine, a powerful antipsychotic drug] brought in by the truckload. They used it as a chemical restraint. Nursing homes back then didn't have a lot of help, so the best help they had was to drug the patients. I knew it wasn't humane, and I fought it from day one."

As Neel got more and more interested in long-term care, the company he started, Institutional Pharmacy Consultants, became a national leader in drug therapy management. In the mid-1990s, according to one survey, patients in IPC-served nursing homes were using drugs at a rate 41 percent lower than the national average. Neel and the pharmacists he trained could lower drug use across the board while improving patient outcomes at the same time.

IPC's business was acquired by a bigger company in 2000, but Neel chafed at being

17

confined to an office in a high-rise building in suburban Atlanta. So at the beginning of the following year, he decided to walk out of the operation he founded and start again from scratch, but vowing this time that he would let nothing get between him and the patients he was trying to help.

So on this Wednesday night in July 2004, Neel is driving to a $30-a-night mom-and-pop motel in rural Georgia that he's stayed in many times before. It's just a stone's throw from a county-owned nursing home Neel counts among his nine institutional clients.

The next morning, at a little after nine, Neel will already be at work there, stationed at a small desk near the nursing director's office. He brings his own office with him: a notebook computer, a portable printer, and a small case of blank forms and printed materials. He knows just about everyone he sees in the facility by name — nurses, patients, family members, and others.

The doctor who serves as the nursing home's medical director, it turns out, doesn't much care for Neel and his approach to the monthly medication reviews mandated by federal law — that many others see as rubber-stamp work. The doctor

18

avoids Neel like the plague and deals with him almost entirely through the nursing staff. (Neel, upon introducing himself for the first time at a meeting of the physicians who work at the nursing home, turned to him and said, "I'm the man who's always pissing you off.")

Throughout the day, Neel will type his medication-related suggestions on a form he designed (printed on pink paper so as to stand out in the patient's medical records) that directs the physician to check a box saying "Accept" or "Reject." This process is the basic building block of what's known in the industry as "drug therapy management" — a series of checks and balances on the prescribing habits of physicians.

The medical director has earned the nickname "Dr. No" because he rejects, almost without exception, Neel's suggestions. He evidently takes umbrage at being second-guessed by a lowly pharmacist — something, Neel says, that's not at all unusual in his profession. He finds the lack of engagement troubling. "He's here once a month," Neel says. "Maybe five minutes per patient. That's all they're required to do."

Neel begins working his way through a tall stack of blue loose-leaf binders that contain patient charts and other medicals.

Each binder is about two inches thick. Today he's reviewing the charts of patients who are taking nine or more prescription medications simultaneously.

It's important on two counts that Neel — or someone like him — review the drug therapies these patients are receiving. First is safety. The risks of adverse drug events increase exponentially with the number of medications "on board," partly because they indicate numerous diseases or other medical problems and provide an opportunity for both drug-disease and drug-drug interactions. Second is cost. "The rule of thumb," Neel says, "is one hundred dollars a drug." That's per patient, per month. Thus, the cost of having a patient on fifteen different medications is $1,500 a month, or $18,000 a year — which means that over-medicating residents can cost the average nursing home (and, in turn, Medicaid and Medicare) hundreds of thousands of dollars a year.

First up today is the chart for a sixty-eight-year-old patient who is on, among many other drugs, nitrofurantoin, an antibiotic that's prescribed for urinary tract infections. Neel enters the man's weight, height, age, and some information from his blood-work into a Casio calculator that's programmed with certain formulas he uses over and over. "His renal clearance is inadequate to clear that drug," Neel says, explaining that toxic levels of the drug will build up in his system because his kidneys aren't as efficient as they used to be. Why, then, would a doctor prescribe it? "Because," Neel says, "it works in young people."

In reviewing the chart of the next patient, a seventy-two-year-old man who'd been admitted to the nursing home for dementia and chronic anemia just two months earlier, Neel notices that the same doctor has put this patient on iron three times a day — a decision, he says, that among other things is bound to make the man's already severe constipation even worse. He winces. "This shows me that he doesn't have any inkling of what he's doing," Neel says. "The only way to get his hemoglobin up is through IV [intravenous] iron or to give him blood." The thought takes Neel down another path. "If you get the iron stores up in his blood," he says, "a lot of the dementia might go away." In his suggestions for the doctor — which, he says, are certain to be rejected — Neel writes a blunt rejoinder to the doctor's choice of treatment: "Oral iron therapy is of no value." Then, noticing that the man is on Benadryl, the brand-name version of the antihistamine diphenhydramine, Neel adds, "No need for use of anticholinergic Benadryl, which also places the patient at high risk for falls." Neel calls the mix of medications he sees on the chart "almost a recipe for falls."

The next chart is for an eighty-nine-year-old woman who was admitted to the home the previous December. She's on thirteen different prescription medications, including Zantac, an acid-suppressing drug that raises an immediate flag for Neel. There are no blood-chemistry tests in her charts, but Neel quickly computes her probable creatinine (renal) clearance at 32.5 cubic centimeters a minute. "This tells me right off the bat she shouldn't be taking it," he says. He then types his suggestion to the doctor: "Zantac dose too high/could lead to 'hepatic shutdown' . . . resulting in serious patient adverse events."

The woman, it turns out, is also on Paxil ("a good drug," he says, "but just not in older people"), for depression and anxiety, and Toprol, a beta-blocker, for high blood pressure. But Toprol, Neel points out, is contraindicated (generally deemed inadvisable) in patients with depression, "and that's the reason she's on the Paxil." Moreover, he says, Paxil's side effects include confusion, dizziness, hypotension (lowered blood pressure), impaired cognition, and vertigo. Little wonder, he says, that the woman has had falls in the nursing home. The doctor's reaction, he points out, was to order a "fall monitor" and "fall protections." "Why not get rid of the cause?" Neel wonders aloud.

He opens the next chart, that of an eighty-two-year-old woman who's on seventeen different medications, including, for type 2 diabetes, a prescription drug called metformin. He's dumbfounded at first, then angry. He reads the suggestion slip he typed out a month and a half earlier: "Patient with serum creatinine clearance less than 60cc/min; use of metformin is contraindicated and places the patient at high risk for lactic acidosis, which is fatal in most cases." What's more, Neel suspects that the patient has been prescribed other drugs that don't get along very well with metformin. "What would be some of the drugs?" he asks rhetorically as he consults a reference guide on his notebook computer. "Well, some of those are on board." They include a beta-blocker; digoxin, a medicine for heart problems; and a twice-daily dose of Zantac. He focuses on his computer screen and types, "Suggestions made to you on

05.25.2004 were rejected. Please reevaluate these completely, since continued therapy at present drug regimen places this patient in serious danger that could lead to death."

And so it goes, over and over and over, throughout the day. Neel says that he almost always sees drugs on the charts that never should be used in geriatric patients, as well as drugs redundantly prescribed for the same condition and drugs that should not be prescribed concurrently.

Neel makes it a habit to lunch in the nursing home cafeteria with the staff (something the doctors rarely if ever do), and he spends much of the time soaking up little details on residents that may prove useful as he reviews their charts. On the way back from the cafeteria, he stops to visit with some of them in their rooms or in the hallway. He seems to make it a point to have some physical contact with each resident — holding one of their hands as he talks, for example, or placing a comforting hand on a shoulder. Later he explains that doctors in the nursing home tend to shun such contact and that a little touch goes a long way in winning the attention, and trust, of residents.

That afternoon, Neel conducts what's called an "in-service" — a kind of seminar, this one on psychoactive drugs — for the nursing home's staff. Despite the thunderstorm raging outside, he has an attentive and seemingly appreciative audience. After the session, he returns to finish reviewing the charts.

A seventy-four-year-old woman with Parkinson's disease has been pacing outside the room where Neel works, and he waves her inside. She wants to ask him about a medicated shampoo that she hasn't used yet partly because the active ingredient is in a separate container and partly because she fears it will interfere in some way with her weekly trip to the beauty parlor. Neel mixes the shampoo on the spot, tells her to use it with a nurse's help that evening, and assures her that she can keep her Friday morning appointment with the hairdresser.

Neel has made yet another friend in the nursing home, which pleases him to no end. "I'm not here," he says, "just to sign charts."

Neel is up early the next morning to check out of the motel and drive to another nursing home about twenty miles south. There, too, he has a combative relationship with the doctor who serves as the facility's medical director. "I don't like a pharmacist telling me what to do," the doctor once complained to the nursing home's administrator, who supports Neel in his role as consulting pharmacist. "Then do it right," the administrator replied.

As soon as Neel arrives, he searches out a seventy-three-year-old male patient who's been there since February 1999. The man, who has advanced Parkinson's, brightens instantly. When Neel first looked at his chart, the man was on 20 milligrams of Zyprexa, an antipsychotic medication, which by any measure is therapeutic overload. He's now down to 2.5 milligrams a day, and soon, Neel says, the daily dose will be even lower. The man's previous symptoms — nonstop yelling, tongue thrusting, "pill rolling" (a parkinsonian tremor that takes the form of a continuous back-and-forth motion of the thumb and fingers) — have all disappeared, and now he sometimes comes to sit next to Neel, without uttering so much as a word, while he works in the nurse's station.

Neel is particularly proud of this case because until recently, the man spent days and nights curled stiffly in a fetal position in his bed. He was all but vegetative. The physician overseeing his treatment told Neel and the nursing staff that the man would never walk again. But walk he now does —

and walk and walk. He visits other residents in their rooms and likes to sit near the main nursing station, the hub of activity. "I gave him his life back," Neel says matter-of-factly, and the man seems to know this too.

One of the problems, as Neel sees it, is that precious few of the three hundred or so doctors who work in the nine facilities he visits specialize in working with geriatric patients. How many do? "Maybe two," Neel says.

"They're not up to date with the physiology of the geriatric patient as it relates to the chemistry of the drugs," he explains. "That's the easiest way to put it."

At a nurse's request, Neel opens the chart of a ninety-seven-year-old woman who has been complaining to the staff about her medications. Her physician has rejected all of Neel's suggestions in the past — including one to discontinue Fosamax, an anti-osteoporosis drug — by checking the "Rejected" box and writing "Patient Stable" underneath. "You aren't going to build bone in the next two or three years," Neel says, and then he writes on a suggestion slip, "At 97 years of age, prognosis for stronger bones is pointless. Please justify why serious risk to this patient does not outweigh benefits."

Next comes the chart of a seventy-six-year-old man who was admitted to the nursing home way back in 1976, when the state's psychiatric institutions were being emptied on a wholesale basis. "He lived in hell," Neel says, referring to the old mental hospitals, "and went to heaven." The man has leukemia and anemia — both, Neel says, the likely result of years and years of being treated with Thorazine, an antipsychotic that left a generation of geriatric patients with disfiguring and irreversible movement disorders.

Next, Neel reviews the chart of a seventy-eight-year-old man who, Neel determined, had been misdiagnosed as a type 2 diabetic by the facility's medical director. "He's on two platelet inhibitors [drugs that are prescribed to prevent blood clots]," Neel points out. "Both do the same thing." What's more, since March he's been taking Megace, a drug that's supposed to stimulate the appetite. Neel notes that the man has had "no weight gain in four months," which, he says, is proof that the drug isn't working. In its place, Neel recommends two ounces of red wine before meals, which he deems to be safer and more effective than Megace.

Neel reviews a few more patient charts before calling it a day, producing more of the pink suggestion slips, each numbered sequentially, as he goes. A little while back, he passed the 300,000 mark.

In the right circumstances, Neel's work saves lots of money — and, perhaps, lots of lives. "There's a lot of resistance to what I do," he says. "I'm still considered a renegade or an off-the-wall kook. But I don't care, I really don't. I know I do good, and I know there are tens of thousands alive because of what I did."

A recent study by the American Society of Consultant Pharmacists found that drug therapy management boosts optimal outcomes by 43 percent and, by preventing medication-related problems, saves $3.6 billion a year. Yet the remaining challenge is staggering. Studies show that for every dollar now spent on medications in nursing facilities, two dollars are spent on treating medication-related problems.

At another nursing home in Georgia, where Neel has known the medical director for about twenty-five years, the success of a collaborative approach is clear. "If I write up a suggestion to paint the nose blue," Neel jokes, "when I go back the next time, the nose is blue." The daily cost for drugs per patient there is down to $6.19, the lowest in Georgia and about half the statewide average. It's a large facility, with 178 beds, but on an average day, 151 residents go to the dining room to eat their meals — an almost unheard-of ratio that speaks to the benefits of appropriate medication levels.

Neel will be back in Griffin before suppertime, where he'll finish the written report that he promised Ruby Gifford before leaving for a weeklong vacation with his wife, children, and grandchildren.

Neel doesn't yet know that Gifford's physician will be angered by her decision to seek his help. As it later happens, the doctor not only refuses to read Neel's seventeen-page report but also asks Gifford to leave the office — and, presumably, not to return.

And so soon Armon Neel will help Ruby Gifford find a new doctor. He is not one to pass the buck. "I've always gotten along well with old people," he says. "They've always been special to me." A mischievous smile breaks out. "And I really like 'em now, 'cause I'm one of 'em."

I wrote these words in the summer of 2004. Some time earlier, Robert Wilson, who was then the editor of the *AARP Bulletin*, had asked me to consider writing a piece for the publication that would look at the idea of getting people in nursing homes off of prescription drugs rather than piling on more of them.

I don't remember exactly how it came to be that the stars aligned in a way that led me one day to call Armon Neel, but they did. I remember our first conversation — with me calling him in Griffin, Georgia, from my office at the AARP in Washington, DC — as if it happened just yesterday. I recall explaining that I was looking for a way to tell the story that my editor had proposed, that I'd been told there were pharmacists who specialized in assessing the appropriateness of a person's medications, and that his name had come to my attention.

"Well, I'm really happy that you called me," I remember Armon Neel telling me, "because I have a message that I want people to hear." He emphasized the word *message* in a way that made me think, almost instantly, that he was exactly the person I'd been looking for. He went on to tell me that he'd devoted most of his career in pharmacy to studying how drugs affected older people, and how drugs often hurt them more than they helped, and how it had nearly always been an uphill battle to get out his message. As we talked more on the phone that day, I realized that this wasn't just a man with a message. This was a man with a mission.

In a week's time, I was on a plane to Atlanta to meet Neel in person and accompany him on his nursing home rounds. I was standing at curbside when I saw his little Miata pull up — he'd described it in some detail as I was making arrangements to come down to Georgia. Out he bounded, with a wide smile and a mop of sandy-white hair made unruly by the top-down drive from Griffin, which is nearly an hour south of Atlanta. After we'd stowed my bag in the Miata's tiny trunk and gotten in the car, Neel handed me a fancy paper bag with a souvenir T-shirt for my daughter and a copy of *The Stuffed Griffin,* a local cookbook, for me. While journalists aren't supposed to accept gifts from the people they write about, I figured that it would be silly in this instance to invoke the rule I had lived and worked by in Washington for so long.

Some hours later, we were in Tifton, Georgia, and in the days ahead, I tagged along as Neel went about his work in some of the nursing homes that were on his "circuit" as a consultant pharmacist back then. Every bit of the way, I felt that I was getting an education of sorts, and I knew this was exactly what Bob Wilson had in mind when he urged me to stop editing for a while and to go back to reporting and writing. I filled a new legal pad with notes as I sat next to Neel and probably asked "Can you spell that for me?" or some variant of it more than I ever have in my life. The drug names and medical terminology nearly overwhelmed me at first, but Armon Neel proved to be a patient and insightful teacher.

In time we circled back to Griffin, a place that retains so much of its 1940s-era look that some of the scenes in the movie *Driving Miss Daisy* were filmed there. The railroad tracks through town run to one side of the historic building that Neel has made into his office, and if you turn right on foot out of the front door, you'll be walking down a street of storefronts that don't seem to have changed a whit in decades. On my first day in Neel's offices, Frank Lindsey, who runs things when Neel is on the road, surprised me by explaining that he'd given up a career in banking to work with the pharmacist he credits with having saved his mother's life. Neel opened his life to me — I met family members, friends, patients — but soon I was heading back to Washington. I had a story to write.

That article, which appeared in the September 2004 issue of the *AARP Bulletin,* struck a pretty powerful chord. The Web site of the American Society of Consultant Pharmacists, which was referenced in the story as a source of additional information, went down momentarily under the weight of inbound traffic. I began getting calls at the AARP virtually every day from people who wanted to reach Neel, and Neel told me that he was getting calls from all over the country. For some years after that, the piece that I wrote for the *Bulletin* still topped its list of best-read — and most-remembered — stories.

The message that Armon Neel wanted people to hear clearly had an audience.

The book you have in your hands is all about that message too: namely, that while prescription drugs can work wonders and save lives, they can also wreak havoc and end lives. This holds especially true for older people, who, on average, are prescribed drugs in greater variety and greater quantity than anyone else.

Most of us do not have much education about the drugs that we and our loved ones take, so this book is mostly a starting point to a different way of looking at the medications we so often use without thinking.

INTRODUCTION:
A PHARMACIST'S JOURNEY

Back in the mid-eighteen hundreds, my great-great-grandfather settled in southeast Mississippi and started a little town that he named Binsville. He owned most of the businesses there, including the cotton gin, the livery stable, and a big three-story building that housed a general store.

In 1889 he added an apothecary, Neel's Pharmacy, and space for each of his three brothers: a doctor, a dentist, and an undertaker. They always used to say that the sign on the front of the building said "Neel Bros. — We Cover You from the Womb to the Tomb." While I never saw a picture of this sign, my relatives swear that it did exist.

As the railroads started to play such an important part in business in the early nineteen hundreds, the entire town was moved three miles east, just across the border with Alabama, and renamed Geiger. The railroad passed right through Geiger and right by Neel's Pharmacy. The pharmacist was my grandfather.

My father came to Atlanta to attend pharmacy school, and after World War II, my parents moved to Griffin, where he opened another Neel's Pharmacy and where my two brothers and I grew up. In school my favorite subject, by far, was chemistry. I loved working alongside my dad in the pharmacy, often compounding the medicines to be dispensed. It always excited me to see the chemistry of the different elements being combined, and I was fascinated by their actions and reactions.

I was very conscious of the different interactions between the patient and pharmacist, as well as the interactions between the patient and the doctor and the doctor and the pharmacist. What I saw, in fact, made a huge impression on me and shaped my future career. When I was accepted to the University of Georgia's School of Pharmacy in 1958, I told my dad that I didn't want to come back to the drugstore and fill prescriptions. He looked at me with no small degree of shock — at least, I think that's what it was.

"What in the hell do you want to do?" he asked. I told him that I saw a big void between the patient and the drug, and that

I wanted to fill that void. So we sat down and talked for several hours about my idea. All the while, he listened patiently and intently. Then he spoke.

"Son, God has given you a vision, and I want you to follow that vision with all my support," he said. "But you will never make a living at it."

After graduating from pharmacy school and finishing my tour of duty with the Army National Guard, I opened an apothecary shop behind the hospital in Griffin. I filled prescriptions, but I also set up a counseling room where I could sit down with patients and develop a drug therapy program to meet their individual needs. I started keeping detailed patient records, which I used to keep up with all of the patients' medical needs. This was in 1963.

Back then it was against the law for a pharmacist to discuss drugs and their effects with a patient. I did it anyway because I knew that it was right and that it was needed. It was not until the late 1980s, when I was asked to help rewrite the Georgia Pharmacy Practice Act, that the law was changed.

In 1966 I changed my apothecary shop into what I called a pharmaceutical center.

There was no merchandise in view, just a waiting area and a reception desk, and then an enclosed pharmacy work area not visible to patients. Around the waiting area were counseling rooms for pharmacist-patient consults. I started educational programs for patients on everything from blood pressure to prenatal care. I was surprised to see how many patients routinely attended these programs and needed information on how to care for themselves and their conditions or illnesses.

In 1967 a close friend of mine who was an administrator of a nursing home asked me to be a consultant for his institution. I declined, explaining that I had my hands full moving forward with my vision for pharmacy care. He kept after me, though, and finally talked me into coming out and visiting his facility. It was a revelation.

Here I saw a new population of very old people for whom the traditional acute-care hospital policies and procedures did not fit at all. I quickly learned that the medications, and the dosing of medications, that worked well in my younger patients often did not work at all in these very old people — and even produced scary results. I could see that there was an urgent and unfilled need to develop the procedures and technology required for providing these patients with appropriate palliative care — that is, care aimed at relieving and preventing their suffering.

All of the nursing home residents had chronic diseases, and often multiple chronic diseases, and we knew that we were not going to be able to cure them. I realized that developing a program to provide the maximum quality of life was the best direction in which to go. Back in those days, we didn't really know exactly *why* many drugs worked in the way that they did, so the package inserts said simply, "Mechanism of action unknown."

So we began a program to research drug therapy outcomes. We had the laboratory to do it, and the patients to help us gather data for acceptable drugs, doses, and predictions in geriatric populations. Throughout the years, we published our findings in medical journals and in other formats to help improve the overall health of all geriatric patients.

But it didn't take long for us to figure out that physicians were not receptive to the idea of pharmacists telling or trying to teach them anything new. Trying to swing physicians around from practicing acute care and into practicing palliative care, we found, was something like trying to turn around an ocean liner. One day I was sitting at my desk, discouraged about the mountain of rejections from doctors, when my dad walked in with a bumper sticker that read, "What's Popular Is Not Always Right . . . What's Right Is Not Always Popular." He handed it to me and said, "Stick this on your car."

I did. And I've always kept another one on my desk to keep me on track whenever things get tough.

We developed the first computer documentation programs for long-term care as well as the nation's first unit-dose drug delivery system — a safer way to dispense and control medications in nursing homes and other institutional settings.

In 1977 I decided to sell my community pharmacy and commit to being a consultant pharmacist. This was a big decision because I had two boys about four years away from college, a house, and all the obligations you get when you are moving along in life, and here I was at thirty-eight years old starting all over again. Well, two months after getting into my new consulting office, it caught on fire and burned to the ground. I lost everything. I was sitting in what was left of one of the chairs with my head in my hands when my dad walked in, patted my shoulder, and handed me a piece of paper that said, "I can do everything through Him who gives me strength" (Philippians 4:13). He patted my shoulder again and said, "Well, what are we going to do?" I looked at him and said, "We're going to clean this mess up and play like it didn't happen." And we did.

My services were needed all over the state, and my practice grew fast. Many times we saw different outcomes with our geriatric patients than were presented in the literature, as there was no requirement by the US Food and Drug Administration that a representative number of patients over sixty-five years of age be included in clinical trials. The studies, we found, were also biased, consistent with which drug companies had paid for them.

And so in 1980 we decided to dedicate $10,000 of our revenue every month to carrying out drug therapy outcome studies on people over age sixty-five. In 1990 we doubled that to $20,000 a month and kept doing it until I sold the consulting firm in 2000. We had grown to more than one hundred employees and a patient base of nearly twenty thousand.

During this time, we developed therapeutic diets exclusively for the geriatric population, programs for treating specific disorders and diseases, and protocols for everything between a facility's front doors and exit lights. We were asked to help write the 1987 Nursing Home Reform Act, a road map to providing quality care for patients in these institutions.

I eat, live, and breathe geriatric drug therapy, but the consulting firm had gotten so big that I couldn't find time to see patients while running the business. Long ago, my dad had given me a little clipping from a column in the *Griffin Daily News* called The Country Parson. I had it framed and put it on my desk. The parson's quote for that day was, "If you are satisfied with where you are, you set your goals too low."

That saying gave me the idea that it might be best to move on and continue working toward my vision in drug therapy management. I had almost filled the void between the drug and the patient, but there was more work to do. I opened a practice devoted exclusively to consulting with outpatients and retained a couple of the nursing homes I had worked in for more than thirty years. They had always been my learning ground.

Ever since then, I have continued to do

research; speak to health care groups and various medical organizations across the United States; spread the message to church groups, civic clubs, and the like; work one-on-one with lots of patients; work with physicians (at least those who will work with me); and teach at various medical, nursing, and pharmacy schools to help make life better for those wonderful old patients.

I'm seventy-three now and still working on the same vision. I have completed more than 400,000 consults. Around fifty thousand saved lives. Dad suggested long ago that I pray every day to make sure my head is on straight and my vision bright. I've always done just that, and this is my prayer:

Oh God, please give me
The *vision* to make the right path
The *wisdom* to teach by example
The *passion* to always bring honor to my
    profession and
The *compassion* to always feel my
    patient's pain.

GOOD-BYE AND GOOD LUCK: HELPING YOURSELF TO BETTER HEALTH

Kenneth Hubbard,* an eighty-year-old retiree, was physically active and mentally alert. One day while shopping at a local mall, his wife urged him to get a cholesterol test. It came in high, so he decided to visit his physician.

Hubbard's doctor looked at the results and without any further tests prescribed atorvastatin (Lipitor), a statin drug, which Hubbard began taking dutifully. About a month later, he was back in his doctor's office, with complaints of joint and muscle pain and problems with his legs twitching at night, making it difficult for him to sleep. (These, in fact, were caused by the drug that Hubbard was taking.) "Well," the physician said, "you're getting on up there and

* The names of patients in this book, occasionally with some identifying details, have been changed for privacy reasons.

probably have a little arthritis and restless leg syndrome." Hubbard left with prescriptions for naproxen, a nonsteroidal anti-inflammatory drug, or NSAID, that he began taking twice daily for arthritis, and pramipexole (Mirapex), a dopamine agonist that he began taking at bedtime for restless leg syndrome.

Soon Hubbard's stomach began to bother him — he was now buying Tums in 160-count containers — and his wife noticed some worrisome changes in his mental state. (Both problems, in fact, were caused by the new drugs.) Hubbard was soon back in his doctor's office, accompanied by his wife, mostly to talk about his newfound confusion, hallucinations, and memory problems. "Well," the internist said, "it isn't unusual for someone of your age to have problems like this" — he walked them through the typical profile of Alzheimer's disease — "so we'll start you on a cholinesterase inhibitor to help slow down the process." They left with a prescription for donepezil (Aricept), which Hubbard began taking the same day.

A month or so later, he was back in his physician's office once again, this time complaining of not being able to play golf, drive his car, or lift his arms above his head, along with constant heartburn and stomach pains and general weakness and dizziness. (These too were all drug effects.) He feared that something was seriously wrong, but the doctor said reassuringly, "All old people have reflux and GI problems. We can stop the stomach discomfort with a proton pump inhibitor." Hubbard left with a prescription for pantoprazole (Protonix).

By now Hubbard was a changed man. He complained of weakness, dizziness (especially when he stood after sitting or lying down), and lethargy. He stopped playing golf and mostly just sat around the house. Hubbard was reluctant to see his physician again, but his wife persuaded him to do so. During the visit, the doctor drew blood to check Hubbard's hemoglobin, the iron-rich protein that carries oxygen from the lungs to the rest of the body. Seeing that the level was low, he started him on ferrous sulfate to build up his iron stores and improve the hemoglobin values. The doctor didn't realize that because ferrous sulfate is acid sensitive, it can't be absorbed in the stomach — and therefore useless — when given with the proton pump inhibitor, and, further, that his patient's problems stemmed from malnutrition and blood loss.

A month later, during a follow-up visit,

Hubbard's physician found lower hemoglobin values, assumed that his patient had a twenty-four-hour virus, and upped the ferrous sulfate to three times a day. He didn't think to check for *Clostridium difficile* diarrhea. (*C. difficile* is a bacterium that can cause difficult-to-treat, life-threatening infections.) That, in fact, was Hubbard's biggest problem, and it was brought on by the pantoprazole. That's also why he was losing blood values and the essential vitamins and nutrients that are needed to sustain life.

Hubbard didn't live to see his physician again. The death certificate showed that he died in his sleep, at eighty, from old age, with Alzheimer's disease as a secondary condition.

In truth, Hubbard was the victim of unneeded medications, beginning with the introduction of the statin drug and culminating in the drug-induced stomach bleeds that ultimately led to his fatal — but unrecognized — internal hemorrhage.

If you think that Kenneth Hubbard's case is an aberration — something that could never happen to you, someone you love, or someone you know — let me assure you that it isn't. There's even a medical term for what happened to him. We call it the "prescription cascade," where the adverse effects of drugs are misdiagnosed as symptoms of another medical problem, resulting in additional prescriptions and additional adverse effects and additional unanticipated drug interactions. As the consequences of the cascade pile up, further mistakes are all but inevitable.

Adverse reactions from prescription drugs are now the fourth-leading cause of death in the United States, after heart disease, cancer, and stroke, and that's not counting the drug-induced deaths that are mistakenly attributed to illness or disease or are otherwise chalked up to natural causes (as in Mr. Hubbard's case). Prescription drugs are estimated to cause at least 100,000 deaths a year, and they injure another 1.5 million people so severely that they require hospitalization.

Older Americans are most at risk. The risk of prescription drug errors is seven times greater for people sixty-five and older than for younger people, according to Medco Health Solutions, a pharmacy benefits manager. While people sixty-five and older account for just 13 percent of the nation's population, they account for more than a third of all reported adverse drug reactions.

Little wonder: many of them are on a mind-numbing and body-numbing array of powerful and often dangerous medications that have been prescribed by doctors who don't fully understand the changing body chemistries of older people.

I am a pharmacist who specializes in geriatric medicine. I consult with older patients and their families about whether they're taking the right prescription drugs in the right doses. I do this because too many older Americans are being prescribed drugs that their bodies can't handle, and, as a result, they're getting sick and dying sooner than they should.

In the pages that follow, I'll explain to you what everyone — doctors, patients, and especially their family members — should keep in mind about how our bodies change with age. I'll show you why these changes need to be taken into account when prescribing medications to older patients, and the catastrophic results that can occur when they're not.

I'll walk you through many of the medications that pose the biggest threats to older people, and if you're a patient or family member, I'll give you specific questions to ask a doctor in order to ensure you or your loved one is getting the right medication in the right dosage. Armed with the information laid out in this book, you'll be able to ask questions in an informed and nonconfrontational way, so that you can maintain a respectful relationship with your doctor.

Older age can be a complicated and tough road to navigate. I speak from experience: I'm seventy-three. But it doesn't need to be made worse with an unnecessary or damaging mix of prescription drugs. Let's face it: we live in a culture in which it's much easier to prescribe a pill to control a symptom than to find out the real source of one's illness. And, unfortunately, the state of our nation's health care system promotes only this quick-fix response to illness — an approach that I call "cookbook medicine."

As a patient and as a consumer, you have every right to defend yourself from these shortcuts as you seek care for yourself and for those you love. I hope this book will help arm you with much of the same information that I have passed along to the many thousands of patients I have consulted with over the years.

I met Kirk Williams in 2006 after taking care of his mother, a retired college professor in her nineties who had been in a nursing home in Blairsville, Georgia, about two hundred miles away from him. A doctor had told him that his mother was dying and that he might want to move her closer to him for the last few months of her life. He moved her into a nursing home that I visit once a month.

I happened to be there the day she arrived, and I reviewed all of her medications — about sixteen drugs. I recommended that all but two of them be stopped, and the doctor and the nursing home, with whom I've had a close working relationship, did so.

A few months later, Mr. Williams came to the nurses' station and asked for the name of the doctor "who saved my mother's life." He explained that his mother had come to the nursing home to die, but that after the doctor had cut out all her medications, she was no longer confused and was "doing great" — to the point where she was able to spend weekends with him and his family. He was astonished, apparently, that his mother's drug bill had been reduced by $1,100 a month.

The nurse at the station that day told Mr. Williams that it wasn't a doctor who'd cut the medications but the nursing home's consultant pharmacist (me). He asked for my telephone number, called, and made an appointment to see me in my office in Griffin.

He drove about two hundred miles to see me, and I reviewed his own drug therapy. At sixty, he was having multiple problems consistent with his type 2 diabetes and cardiovascular disease (he'd had a heart attack a few years back). He complained of his hands, feet, and fingers always tingling, feeling numb, or burning, sometimes with sharp pains. He was feeling so weak and fatigued that he couldn't exercise and was having dizzy spells in the morning and during the night when he'd get up to go to the bathroom. He was also having frequent headaches.

A little while later, I gave Mr. Williams my report, which ran to twenty-three pages and included recommendations for changes in his drug therapy. At the top of the list was discontinuing metformin (brand name, Glucophage), a drug used to treat diabetes that shouldn't have been prescribed in the first place because of his impaired renal function (as shown by his low creatinine clearance), and replacing it with another antidiabetic drug. I could easily tell that his fatigue and dizziness were consistent with prolonged hypoglycemia, or low blood sugar, and that one of the blood pressure medications prescribed to him — carvedilol (Coreg), a beta-blocker that doubles as an alpha-blocker — was only making things worse. In addition to exacerbating his hypoglycemia, it was also, in all likelihood, responsible for his peripheral vascular disease and, most of all, the symptoms of Raynaud's disease (the numbness and tingling in his extremities). I recommended the use of diltiazem (Cardizem), a benzothiazepine calcium channel blocker, instead.

Mr. Williams later told me that his cardiologist, on being presented with my recommendations, became visibly enraged, saying that he was going to report me to the state for practicing medicine without a license. And his family physician, who had him on $600 to $700 a month of "nutraceuticals" — food-based dietary supplements and other products — that she was selling him out of her office, had a milder but similar reaction. Both doctors refused to consider any of my recommendations.

Eventually, with my help, Mr. Williams found a physician who agreed with my recommendations and, over a period of weeks, implemented all of them. A few months later, Mr. Williams was back in his cardiologist's office for a follow-up and mentioned how much better he felt. The cardiologist responded by telling Mr. Williams that he was going to die and that his bloodwork would prove it by showing how much his cardiac enzymes had deteriorated as a result of my recommendations.

As it turned out, Mr. Williams's cardiac enzymes looked better than they had since his heart attack. His bank account was looking a lot better too. He was saving around $1,100 a month from all the prescription drugs and expensive vitamin preparations that we'd stopped.

For every patient like Kirk Williams that I've been able to help over the years, I know that there are countless others who never even realize that they're being mismedicated or overmedicated. I hope that for at least some of them, this book will be a wake-up call.

THINGS CHANGE: OUR AGING BODIES

On meeting patients for the first time, I often tell them that all of us age at exactly the same rate: one day at a time. There's not a whole lot we can do about it except to take the best care of ourselves that we possibly can and try to make the smartest choices we can when life throws us a curveball.

But along the way, we need to know that our bodies are constantly changing as we age. Some of the changes we can actually see: skin that's not as smooth or elastic as it used to be, for example, or hair that's thinning or going gray. Some of the changes we can feel: joints that are stiffer or creakier, or muscles that ache in ways they never used to. And some of the changes — mostly having to do with our body chemistry — we can't see or feel at all.

Our bodies age slowly. A lot of different forces come into play: genetics, socioeconomic and environmental factors, life events, and traumas of all kinds, including stresses, illnesses, injuries, and diseases.

As we age, we experience sensory changes, including declines in sight and peripheral vision, hearing, smell, and taste. We also experience structural changes, such as the loss of lean body mass (muscle) — which leads to a slowing down of our metabolic rate — and the loss of bone density. And we also experience changes in most of our vital organs.

In this book, you'll be reading a lot about the liver and kidneys, because those are the vital organs that break down drugs and eliminate them from our bodies. These organs change as we age, which has huge implications for nearly everything we put in our bodies: food, vitamins, minerals, alcohol, prescription drugs, over-the-counter medications, you name it.

Let's start with the bean-shaped kidneys. They're the most important filters in our body, cleaning the blood of the waste products generated by our normal metabolic processes. The kidneys also help maintain our body fluids and electrolytes (such as sodium and potassium) at normal levels.

Beginning at the age of thirty, however,

we lose 1 percent of our kidney (renal) function — on average — with each passing year. That means, as a rule of thumb, that the average eighty-year-old has lost half of his or her renal function. An older person's kidneys simply aren't going to process and excrete drugs the way a younger person's kidneys do.

Fortunately, our kidneys are remarkable organs that start out with more capacity than they need. This means that even older kidneys working below "full capacity" can take care of most of the jobs we throw at them. (What's more, some people don't lose all that much kidney function as they grow older.) And because we lose muscle mass at roughly the same rate as we lose renal function, our kidneys are generally able to support our basic body functions well enough for us not to notice that they're not as efficient as they once were.

Unfortunately, however, older kidneys are slower to respond to stresses from disease and other factors. The drugs that we put in our bodies are one of the chief environmental stresses on the kidneys. And because we tend to use drugs, or use *more* drugs, to treat illnesses and diseases, older kidneys tend to get a double whammy in these circumstances.

Our liver chemistry can change dramatically with age too. The liver carries out more than five hundred complex — and essential — functions, from making the enzymes and proteins responsible for most of the chemical reactions in our bodies to clearing our blood of waste products, drugs, and other toxins. Beginning at about age twenty for women and about age twenty-five for men, as the blood supply to the liver gradually declines, we lose 0.3 percent to 1.5 percent of our liver function each year. The blood flow not only brings oxygen and nutrients into the liver but also carries out metabolites (waste products) and toxins.

Our liver actually shrinks and becomes harder as we age. The average weight of a ninety-year-old's liver is about half (51.8 percent) that of a thirty-year-old's.

Some liver chemicals and enzymes that are essential for breaking down many medications also disappear gradually as we grow older. Older people are more susceptible to infections, for example, because our livers aren't as efficient in performing an important immune function — filtering microorganisms out of the nutrients gathered from the digestive tract — as they used to be.

Over time, these two elements — the diminishing blood flow to the liver and the gradual loss of chemicals and enzymes — reduce the liver's ability to repair damage from inflammation caused by viruses, alcohol, or chemicals, including drugs.

A CHEMISTRY LESSON

If chemistry wasn't one of your favorite subjects in school, you may well be inclined to skip over this section. But I'd urge you to stick with this little lesson, as it will help you understand some of the basic calculations used to determine how your liver and kidneys react to drugs.

We'll start with creatinine clearance tests, which tell how well your kidneys are working. They do this by measuring the level of the waste product creatinine in your blood and urine. Creatinine, a by-product of basic metabolism, is filtered out of your blood by the kidneys and then passed out of your body in urine. Because your body makes creatinine at a steady rate (it's not affected by diet or by normal physical activities), measuring it is one of the most useful tools we have at our disposal. As your renal function declines, the level of creatinine in your urine goes down; and because your kidneys aren't flushing it out as efficiently as they used to, the level in your blood goes up.

Calculating a patient's creatinine clearance thus helps us to determine how much time it will take for a particular drug, in a particular dose, to be excreted from the body. And in cases where the kidneys are unable to process and excrete a drug at least as quickly as it is ingested, the creatinine clearance calculation helps us to estimate at what rate the "excess" drug will build up in the body — to potentially toxic, even life-threatening, levels.

Most laboratory reports contain a creatinine clearance (CrCl) calculation that's been derived by using a formula known as MDRD, which stands for Modified Diet in Renal Disease. This formula was developed for a 1999 study of the role of diet in kidney disease and was based on the standard measurement of serum creatinine used by the world-renowned Cleveland Clinic. While the MDRD formula has been validated in other clinical studies of younger patients with chronic renal disease, it is totally deceptive for figuring out the creatinine clearance of patients who are fifty years of age or older. This distinction is important in clinical practice because age-related renal impairment is not the same as chronic renal disease, which can have many different causes.

The most accurate formula for quickly

calculating creatinine clearance in older patients is known as the Cockcroft-Gault equation, which is named after the scientists who first published the formula in 1976. It's more accurate than the MDRD formula because it takes muscle mass into account. I began using this pharmacokinetics formula shortly after it was first presented and continue to use it today.

The most accurate way of all to determine a patient's creatinine clearance, at least in theory, is to collect his or her urine over a twenty-four-hour period and then analyze the amount of creatinine in the sample. The medication therapy consulting firm that I founded used to routinely check the accuracy of the Cockcroft-Gault equation against urine sample results, and after thousands of such comparisons, we found it to be about 95 percent accurate.

A few years ago, I was speaking to a group of physicians on the topic of drug therapy in the older patient. As part of my talk, I mentioned that nitrofurantoin (brand name, Macrobid), an antibiotic that's commonly used to treat urinary tract infections, is one of the drugs that shouldn't be prescribed to older people, as their kidneys typically lack the ability to excrete it, and the consequent drug buildup can lead to many serious adverse events. I explained that an older patient would have to have a creatinine clearance of at least 80 cubic centimeters per minute to tolerate the drug.

A physician in the audience stopped me, saying that he thought Macrobid was good for all patients with urinary tract infections and that he'd never been told about creatinine clearance and the role it plays in determining whether particular drugs are appropriate for older people. Several other physicians agreed. "Well, the culture and sensitivity reports from the lab show that the infection is sensitive to the drug," one of them asked, "so why can't you use it?"

"The drug may be very effective in killing off the bacteria," I replied, "but if the body can't tolerate the drug, then you can kill the patient while you are killing off the infection." There were bewildered looks in the audience. "You have to use drugs that not only are effective against the bacteria," I said, "but that also will be consumed and excreted in an appropriate time period to ensure that the patient gets well."

Over the years, I have had many experiences like this, and I always come away from them alarmed. Little wonder that many older people have such serious health problems.

■ ■ ■ ■

If you study geriatrics, at some point you'll hear about the "basic rule": namely, that by age seventy, the body's organ functions will have diminished to about half their peak levels. The rule is said to apply across the board, from pulmonary function and cardiac output to liver and kidney functions. On top of this, you can add losses of function from disease and disability.

Similarly, our ability to engage in physical activity begins to change at around age fifty. From a physiological standpoint, multiple factors contribute to the gradual deterioration of the body's oxygen delivery systems: decreased elasticity in the chest wall (making it more difficult for the body to obtain the oxygen needed for exercise), lower ventilation-to-perfusion ratios (making it more difficult for the lungs to oxygenate blood), and decreased blood output from the heart (making it more difficult for skeletal muscles to get oxygen). Add to this an actual decrease in skeletal muscle mass.

Aging also brings changes in weight and body composition. Typically, we tend to gain weight up until the age of about sixty, at which point we gradually lose weight. The ratio of lean muscle mass to body fat declines steadily throughout old age.

These age-related changes in our bodies all have important implications for drug therapy, both in the choice of medications and in the formulation of appropriate dosages. In addition to the basic principle we've already covered — that, on the whole, the aging body processes and eliminates most drugs less efficiently, leaving it more vulnerable to toxic accumulations of the medications — there's the fact that older people take more drugs than younger people do. And the chance of two or more medications causing problems as they interact in the body increases with each drug added into the mix.

You've already learned a little bit about pharmacokinetics, which may be defined simply as what the body does to a drug. As pharmacotherapists, we study how a drug is absorbed and distributed in the body (in other words, its mechanism of action), the rate and duration of the drug's desired therapeutic effect, the process by which the body metabolizes the drug (breaks it down chemically), and how the metabolites of the drug affect the body and exit from it. We remember these four processes — absorption, distribution, metabolism, and excretion — with the acronym ADME. Each of these pharmacokinetic processes changes in older patients and has important implications for drug therapy.

Absorption. In and of itself, the aging process has little to no effect on drug absorption. Certain chronic diseases, however, can cause drug absorption problems.

Distribution. Most medications are distributed either to fat or to water within the body. As older people have a higher percentage of body fat than younger people (25 percent to 30 percent more, on average), fat-soluble medications typically stay in their bodies much longer.

Because most of the anesthetic drugs used during surgery are fat soluble, for example, they can remain lodged in the body's fat cells for quite a long time, leaving older patients acting confused or even demented — sometimes for up to several months after an operation. The drugs will eventually dissipate from the fat cells, but the general rule is that the longer the surgery, the longer the recovery time.

As the percentage of body fat in an older

person increases, there's a corresponding decrease in the percentage of his or her body consisting of water. In older persons, this typically means that blood levels of water-soluble medications will be higher than would be expected otherwise. Digoxin (Lanoxin), a drug used to treat congestive heart failure and the associated symptom of shortness of breath, is a classic example. In drugs with narrow therapeutic windows, there's not much room between a dose needed to be effective and a dose that could be toxic. Despite its narrow therapeutic window and potential fatal toxicity, digoxin is one of the drugs most widely prescribed to older people. But doctors often don't recognize digoxin toxicity in older patients because some of its markers — cognitive changes, blurred vision, and abnormal heart rhythms (arrhythmia) — aren't typically seen in younger people and are consistent with numerous other conditions related to aging.

Finally, diseases that reduce blood levels of the protein albumin are more common in older people and complicate the use of such heavily protein-bound drugs (medications that must latch on to plasma proteins to circulate through the blood) as warfarin (Coumadin), an anticoagulant.

Patients with low albumin levels can't bind as much of the warfarin, allowing it to remain in an active form and build up to toxic levels. This can lead to life-threatening bleeding and brain hemorrhages.

Metabolism. In addition to the general decline in liver function that's associated with aging, in an older person, the major enzymatic system by which the liver metabolizes medications — the cytochrome P450 system, or CYP — is saturated more rapidly, leaving it unable to metabolize medications as efficiently as it once did. A dose of the antianxiety drug diazepam (Valium), for example, may pose no problems for a young person, but give it to an older person, and unwanted effects begin to mount almost instantly. In an older person, diazepam's half-life — roughly, the time it takes for half the drug to be eliminated from the body — is ninety-six hours. Because medications continue to accumulate for six half-lives (at which point the amount of drug entering the body equals the amount being excreted), diazepam, if taken daily, will continue to accumulate in the body for nearly three weeks. That's why patients who leave a hospital on diazepam are headed for trouble. A couple of weeks later, they are likely to be dazed, confused, and all but unable to get out of bed. If they do make it out of bed, they're likely to become dizzy and fall.

Excretion. In addition to the general decline in renal function that's associated with aging, the kidneys can also become less efficient because of chronic diseases such as congestive heart failure or diabetes mellitus, as well as conditions such as dehydration and low blood pressure. Particular care must be taken with drugs known to cause nephrotoxicity (the poisoning of kidney cells), including NSAIDs, ACE inhibitors, and certain antibiotics.

YOUR DRUGS, YOUR BODY

Now for a short lesson in pharmacodynamics, which may be defined simply as what a drug does to the body. (It's the flip side of *pharmacokinetics*.) This is what happens from a pharmacologic standpoint when the effects of one drug are influenced or altered by the effects of a second drug.

As we get older, we tend to be more sensitive to most medications. This is especially true for drugs that affect the central nervous system, particularly those with anticholinergic properties. By blocking the effects of acetylcholine — a neurotransmitter

69

(chemical messenger) associated with muscle activation, learning, and memory — anticholinergic drugs can cause constipation, difficulty urinating, blurred vision, confusion, and short-term memory problems, and other adverse effects.

Here's an example. A single 30 milligram dose of flurazepam (Dalmane), one of the most widely prescribed sleeping pills, will cause measurable side effects such as unsteadiness, dizziness, and light-headedness in nearly half of people over sixty who take the drug; the same drug at the same dose will cause measurable side effects in only 5 percent to 10 percent of younger people.

Pharmacotherapists look for three different types of drug-drug interactions:

Additive. This is where the side effects of two or more drugs are amplified because they are administered at the same time. Take one drug like zolpidem (Ambien) for insomnia and another like lorazepam (Ativan) for anxiety, and the additive effects will be compounded, with lethargy, falls, respiratory suppression, and dementia-like symptoms at the top of the list.

Synergistic. This is where two or more drugs interact in ways that enhance or magnify their total effect. Taking acetaminophen (Tylenol) for pain in combination with a dose of tramadol (Ultram), for example, may increase the overall analgesic effects. This can be a beneficial action.

Antagonistic. This is where two or more drugs produce an effect that is less than what the drugs would exert working alone. In my clinical practice, for example, I frequently see donepezil (Aricept), a drug used to treat dementia, prescribed at the same time as oxybutynin (Ditropan), a medication for managing the symptoms of an overactive bladder. In this case, a drug with cholinergic properties (Aricept) is, from a therapeutic standpoint, basically canceling out a drug with anticholinergic properties (Ditropan).

These interactions can occur in people of any age, but in older patients they can lead to some very serious adverse events. When I tell new patients that one or more of the drugs they're taking aren't appropriate for an older person and suggest stopping it, I often hear something like, "Well, I've been taking this drug for forty years, and it hasn't caused any problems." As it turns out, it *has* caused problems; the person just hasn't connected them with the drug.

In a case like this, I have to explain that the reason a patient is now having cardiac arrhythmias and elevated eye pressure that could be glaucoma *and* indigestion and acid reflux is, in all likelihood, the drug that "hasn't caused any problems."

Back when the patient started taking the drug — amitriptyline (Elavil), a tricyclic antidepressant — at the age of twenty-six, every organ system in his or her body was functioning at peak efficiency. But as the years ticked off, the adverse effects of the drug slowly but steadily crept up on the patient. He certainly feels them now but has never associated them with the Elavil because they weren't there from the get-go. But the proof positive is that when you stop the drug, everything returns to normal.

Another patient explains that he's been taking ibuprofen (Motrin) for neck pain for more than thirty years — as it happens, ever since the Upjohn Company put it on the market in 1974. "I take just four pills a day," he tells me. "They made it where you can buy it without a prescription, so I figure it must be safe."

But he figured wrong. He has blood in his stool, a critically low platelet count, and an Hgb (hemoglobin) of 8.8, which means he is bleeding inside. This could have happened when he was younger, but he was lucky. In any event, his GI system can no longer tolerate this kind of NSAID-induced punishment, and his long love affair with Motrin is over.

Soon he'll be on an analgesic instead of an NSAID for his pain, but he needs to go to the emergency room first, where he receives two units of blood. In reasonably short order, a combination of tramadol and acetaminophen at bedtime will resolve the patient's neck problem, stop the bleeding, and get him back on the golf course. But it was a closer call than he ever could have imagined.

"What do you mean the Dramamine is the problem?" another patient asks me. "Dr. Jones prescribed it for me back in the seventies because sometimes I got seasick fishing from my bass boat."

As he tells me all about it, I'm sure that the drug worked well enough for many years. But right now I'm trying to figure out why he fell out of his bass boat yesterday while fishing with a friend. "I don't know," he says. "I just leaned over to open my tackle box and couldn't stop."

The good news, I tell him, is that he's healthy at the age of seventy-eight and can do most of the things he wants to. The bad news (which won't turn out to be bad at all) is that he can no longer take Dramamine — or any other anticholinergic drug, for that matter. "I bet you don't even need it anymore," I tell him. "Why don't you try getting along without it next time?" Within a week, I hear that our little experiment was a success, and ever since then, his boat has been a drug-free zone.

There's nothing wrong with getting old, and, as a matter of fact, there are a lot of great things that can come your way. At seventy-three, I find something to love about every day and probably have more fun than I did when I was half my age. I do nearly all the things I've always liked to do: ride my bike, take my sports car on road rallies, go deep-sea fishing with my sons, play with my grandchildren at home and at our beach house, and work at exactly what I always dreamed of doing.

There are a few things I don't do anymore: I stopped waterskiing quite a few years ago and snow skiing some time after that, for example. But I pay attention to what goes into my body and supplement my diet with the vitamins and nutrients that I either don't make anymore or can't absorb from food anymore.

I enjoy life so much that I try not to waste

a minute of it . . . unless I'm wasting it on something good. Or, as Maurice Chevalier, the French singer and actor who lived to be eighty-three, once said, "Old age isn't so bad when you consider the alternative."

It's important to understand that you can't turn around the aging process, although many people try. All of the claims for "age reversal" medications, dietary supplements, herbs, and the like are just that: claims. The manufacturers and marketers of these products rake in billions of dollars from gullible older people who are eager, or even desperate, to reclaim their youth. They eventually learn what you should accept right here, right now: you're not going to return to the "youthful you" ever again.

When it comes to aging, my philosophy is a simple one: just be thankful that you are here and can enjoy being with your loved ones, playing with your friends, continuing to work for the goals that you set many years ago, and growing older gracefully. Many of those fountain-of-youth products can actually make you age faster and cause cognitive problems that may be irreversible. Some of them, especially when taken with other medications for chronic conditions that you have, may increase your risk of bleeding or, at the opposite end of the spectrum, increase your risk of blood clots, which can cause you to die of a heart attack or a stroke.

Once you hit sixty, if not earlier, it's really important that you work with doctors and other health care professionals who understand the idiosyncrasies of your age group: how your body is changing with age, why certain drugs should be ruled out because of your age and related factors, and what risk factors have entered the equation. The goal, especially if you have any kind of chronic medical condition, is a well-thought-out drug management program that's aimed, day in and day out, at improving your health and quality of life.

As an older adult, you certainly don't want to be seeing a doctor or other health care professional who doesn't understand that you metabolize and eliminate drugs differently from someone ten or twenty or thirty or forty years younger than you. What I call "cookbook medicine" — a doctor prescribing a drug at a certain dose based on the results of a test and a set of practice guidelines — won't work very well for you. (The practice guidelines might even come from a nonprofit organization like the National Osteoporosis Foundation, which is bankrolled largely by drug manufacturers.) You need someone with the skill and time to find out what's causing your problem instead of just addressing it — and each successive problem — with a prescription drug.

PILING ON:
THE PERILS OF POLYPHARMACY

I met Paul Dugan in 2007 when he and his daughter traveled down to Griffin from Emmaus, Pennsylvania, to see if I might be able to help him. I could tell right away, on meeting Mr. Dugan, that he was still sharp as a tack at eighty-four, though maybe in a bit of a fog from being overmedicated.

As his daughter listened and added a few details here and there, Mr. Dugan told me that he was having muscle spasms and muscle pain all over his body. He complained of weakness and fatigue, and his daughter mentioned that lately he often fell asleep in the middle of conversations. His arthritis was bothering him, he said, and he was having lots of stomach problems. He'd been hospitalized at least twice for chest pains.

At the time of our meeting, Mr. Dugan was on twenty-two different prescription medications. As I looked through his medical records, I could see that most of them had been prescribed after he'd been put on the statin drug atorvastatin (Lipitor) in 2002. As I looked at entry after entry, it was clear to me that he had experienced a cascade of health troubles that had brought him much discomfort, multiple hospitalizations and coronary catheterizations, blood loss, and a layering on of additional prescription drugs that had caused his health to deteriorate even further — and, in fact, placed him at high risk for a fatal episode.

Almost immediately after he'd been started on Lipitor in 2002, Mr. Dugan began experiencing more arthritis pain, shoulder pain, leg cramps, and general aches and pains. His doctor's response, I could see from the records, was to start him on pentoxifylline (Trental), which is supposed to improve blood flow in patients with circulation problems, and valdecoxib (Bextra), a relatively new NSAID (nonsteroidal anti-inflammatory drug) that was selling like hotcakes despite the fact that in 2001 the FDA had deemed it "not approvable" for the management of acute pain. The latter drug relieved his pain a little bit, but soon, by virtue of the gastrointestinal toxicity that's a trademark of all NSAIDs, it led to slow GI bleeds. He was then put on the corticosteroid prednisone (Deltasone), presumably to treat his arthritis and muscle pain, but it apparently provided little benefit.

In early 2003 Mr. Dugan was admitted to the hospital with chest pains. At that point, a nitrate called isosorbide (Imdur) was added for angina (the temporary chest discomfort that comes when the heart isn't getting enough blood), along with clopidogrel (Plavix), a blood-clotting inhibitor. During this time, he had bilateral cataract surgery, which was successful and improved his vision dramatically.

That summer, Mr. Dugan complained of being weak, dizzy, and nauseated, and by November, he was back in the hospital, this time with a severe GI bleed. He was put on pantoprazole (Protonix), a proton pump inhibitor that tamps down the secretion of stomach acid, and taken off the prednisone. A little while later, the Bextra, Imdur, and Plavix were removed from his regimen and two blood pressure drugs were added: metoprolol (Toprol), a beta-blocker, and a fixed-dose combination of an ARB and hydrochlorothiazide (a type of diuretic, or "water pill"). He was prescribed ultrasound treatments for his arthritis and cramps.

In 2004, with Mr. Dugan complaining

that the arthritis was all over his body, his doctor prescribed an oxycodone-acetaminophen combination pain drug to be taken throughout the day and at bedtime. When repeated laboratory tests failed to identify arthritis, the diagnosis changed to lupus, an autoimmune disorder, and Mr. Dugan was prescribed extended-release venlafaxine (Effexor XR), an antidepressant.

Shortly after that, Mr. Dugan was admitted to the hospital emergency room for an episode that was diagnosed as an atrial fibrillation, which had converted (corrected itself) on the way to the hospital. At that point, his doctors (1) placed him on clonidine (Catapres), an alpha-adrenergic agonist used to treat high blood pressure; (2) put him back on Toprol; (3) ordered a magnetic resonance imaging (MRI) scan, which diagnosed a torn rotator cuff; and (4) discharged him from the hospital.

In a few months, Mr. Dugan was admitted to the hospital with dangerously low blood pressure and was again treated for angina. Another coronary catheterization was ordered and another stent added. With his leg cramps more severe, a diagnosis of restless leg syndrome was added. Chest X-rays revealed no problems.

In early 2006 Mr. Dugan began having

episodes of severe diarrhea, along with anemia and more cramps and shoulder pains. He gave up golf. His records for the following months revealed more hospitalizations, coronary catheterizations, EKGs, X-rays, symptomatic heart problems, angina, and erratic blood pressures and no relief.

That's when Mr. Dugan and his daughter came down from Pennsylvania to see me. Three years earlier, one of them had apparently read the profile of me in the *AARP Bulletin* and saved the article — or perhaps just my name — for future reference.

Even today, as I look back at his drug therapy throughout this nearly six-year ordeal, I shake my head and wonder how everyone overlooked the obvious side effects precipitated by the Lipitor — the very first drug prescribed for him — which started appearing within a month. The ensuing cascade — the medications ordered to treat the symptoms of the adverse events from statin use and the awful problems that these additional drugs caused — leaves me as stupefied today as the day I first met Mr. Dugan. The severe anemia that was so evident to me had been identified seven months earlier, yet no drug changes had been made, nor were there any attempts to get his dangerously low CBC (complete blood count) values up. The most important CBC values are RBC and WBC (red and white blood cell counts), GR# (granulocyte count), Hb (hemoglobin count), and Plt (platelet count).

He was on multiple blood thinners, aspirin, Plavix, Trental, and vitamin E. He was on a proton pump inhibitor that had pushed his gastric acid pH to such a basic state that his potential risk of *C. difficile* diarrhea — which he'd experienced in the past — was unacceptably high, and the drug-induced loss of folate and vitamin B_{12} further inhibited his chances of getting well.

Additionally, at the time I met Mr. Dugan, he was taking piroxicam (Feldene), the most powerful and dangerous NSAID, which is totally contraindicated in the geriatric patient. All this, especially when viewed against the backdrop of his previous GI bleeds, left him vulnerable to a fatal GI hemorrhage at any time.

In my opinion, the arthritis, chest pain, muscle pain (myalgia), and neuropathic pain (nerve pain) were probably adverse effects from the Lipitor. The subsequent drug therapy mostly just made things worse.

On the day that he first came to my office, I calculated Mr. Dugan's creatinine clearance (CrCl) at 39 cc/min (cubic centimeters per minute), which made many of the drugs prescribed to him contraindicated. His impaired kidney function, as reflected in his CrCl level, undoubtedly was responsible for many of the serious adverse episodes he had experienced. His seesawing blood pressure was surely due to the many different antihypertensives prescribed, the alpha-blocker agents used to control his blood pressure, and the tamsulosin (Flomax) — an alpha-blocker — prescribed for his BPH (benign prostatic hyperplasia), better known as an enlarged prostate. And his excessive use of acetaminophen — in excess of 3,000 milligrams a day — put him at very high risk of hepatotoxicity, or drug-induced liver damage.

Mr. Dugan's determination to get well, I think, had a lot to do with his role as the sole caregiver for his wife, who had dementia. "His devotion and dedication to making sure she is taken care of is paramount in his mind," I wrote in my notes at the time, going on to say, "I truly believe that if we can remove these drugs and allow the body to heal itself that his playing golf again is not an unrealistic goal. I know that consistent with the youthful dexterity he displays, his return to good health is a very strong possibility."

In my notes, I also described Mr. Dugan as a casualty of "the polypharmacy war."

Paul Dugan is doing well these days — as I write this, he just celebrated his eighty-eighth birthday — but the war he survived rages on, claiming new victims by the day.

Polypharmacy — meaning "many drugs" — refers to problems that can occur when someone takes multiple medications. It is a national epidemic. It's responsible for up to 28 percent of all hospital admissions, studies show, and would rank as the fifth-leading cause of death in the United States if it were so classified.

Polypharmacy affects mostly older people and poses special — often life-threatening — problems for them. People sixty-five and older make up about 12 percent of the US population but account for nearly 34 percent of all prescriptions written. At any given time, the average older American is taking four or five prescription drugs and at least two over-the-counter medications, and it's not at all unusual for people in nursing homes or other long-term care facilities — or for people still living at home with several concurrent medical conditions — to be taking many, many more than that.

Paul Dugan was taking twenty-two medications at the time he first came to me, and that's pretty much par for the course in my practice. People on that many drugs often feel so weighed down by them, feel so unlike their former selves, that they — or a loved one — finally get to the point where they reach out for help.

You don't have to be a doctor or a pharmacist to see that polypharmacy presents a nearly endless array of dangers for older people. How is it conceivable that ten, twenty, thirty, or even forty prescription drugs could be safe and appropriate for a single patient? When do these drugs, in combination, become toxic? Which of the drugs pushes the body over the precipice of chemical overload? And at what point do the drugs, in combination, become more dangerous to a patient than the conditions they are intended to treat?

These questions are all important because, as a medical certainty, the more drugs a person takes, the higher the risk of adverse interactions.

Many of the case studies in this book show exactly how drugs layered on top of drugs — the former often prescribed to treat the side effects of the latter — can set off a potentially fatal cascade of problems. I often think of this irresponsible, even reckless, type of drug layering to be nothing short of malpractice.

Too many of the nation's doctors and other health care practitioners really don't know what they're doing when they prescribe drugs to older patients. And we have nowhere near as many consultant pharmacists — people who are trained to spot life-destroying drug combinations — as we need to have. As I see it from my admittedly biased perspective, they are an older person's last line of defense when it comes to ill-conceived drug therapy.

As you may already have learned from this book, older Americans often lack the body chemistry that's needed to break down drugs, distribute them throughout the body, and eliminate them promptly. Yet many of them are on five or more medications. Let me tell you: if that describes you, the sixth prescription is probably there to deal with problems caused by the other five.

Nearly every day, I see patients who are taking so many prescription drugs, over-the-counter medications, and vitamins and other dietary supplements that they can't even keep track of them all. Some, in our first consultation, even joke about not knowing how many drugs they're on or why, exactly, many of them were prescribed.

It's not a laughing matter. With each drug you add on top of the first one, the risk of a dangerous drug interaction increases. The estimated incidence of such interactions, in fact, rises from 6 percent in individuals who take two medications a day to as high as 50 percent in those who take five medications a day. The risk increases exponentially; soon after five medications a day, you hit the 100 percent risk threshold.

For many older people, part of the problem is that they're seeing different doctors for different health issues. In fact, studies have shown that an older person's risk of an inappropriate drug combination is directly related to the number of different physicians prescribing drugs for him or her. And many older people make matters worse by filling their prescriptions at different pharmacies. In such cases, there may be no one pharmacist or other health care professional who sees all the different medications they're taking and can screen them for potentially dangerous combinations.

It requires a lot of knowledge too — and sophisticated, up-to-date computer software — to identify potentially dangerous drug interactions. A person taking 10 medications, for example, has 44 possible drug-drug interactions that need to be analyzed; a patient taking 15 medications has 104 such possible interactions.

That's why many people come to see me on their own, and why doctors with whom I have a collaborative relationship often send their patients to me. Take, for example, Katie Cooper, who was referred to me in 2006 by a doctor in Griffin. She'd come to him because, after years of being treated by a local cardiologist, she could no longer stand up on her own.

Guided by her daughter, Mrs. Cooper hobbled into my office, tightly clutching the top rails of a walker. At eighty-three, she was on twenty-one different medications. She was confused and forgetful, incontinent, and very depressed, and she lived with her daughter because she could no longer care for herself.

I found Mrs. Cooper to be very bright, alert, and pleasant but with a high degree of anxiety and depression over her physical condition. She complained of recent falls — including one in the shower — and of feeling weak and lethargic, among quite a few other problems. She was especially upset about losing her driving privileges because of the confusion and falls.

I could see immediately that Mrs. Cooper was taking too many blood pressure drugs. The overmedication had left her with an average a.m. blood pressure of 105/57 and a pulse of 60, and an average p.m. blood pressure of 99/55 and a pulse of 64. It amazed me that she hadn't fallen more often with blood pressures in this very low range. She was also experiencing orthostatic hypotension — a sudden drop in blood pressure every time she stood up, leaned over, or moved about quickly — clearly why she was feeling so weak and dizzy.

Mrs. Cooper had also been prescribed temazepam (Restoril), a benzodiazepine tranquilizer, to help her sleep. The use of this drug at 30 milligram doses is totally contraindicated in older patients, as they lack the liver enzymes needed to break down the drug and over time develop a strong psychological and physiological dependence on it. As the residual drug accumulates in the body, it causes unsteadiness, dizziness, and falls — all problems that Mrs. Cooper had been experiencing.

Katie's new doctor followed the recommendations in my thirty-six-page report to the letter. By the time of her follow-up visit with me a couple of months later, her total drug costs had been reduced by more than

$1,000 a month. She arrived at my office by herself, without a walker. As it turned out, she had been able to drive herself there.

I'll never forget how reenergized and cute Mrs. Cooper was on this visit. She wanted to know the name of the male physician's assistant who'd drawn her blood for the lab test I'd requested. "Boy," she told me, "he was so good-looking that if I were sixty years younger, I would have given him my phone number."

"Girl," I replied, "we need to calm you down some before you get into trouble."

Mrs. Cooper was feeling so much better and was so longing for her independence again that she moved out of her daughter's home and now lives in a retirement community in central Florida, where she has a large circle of new friends, drives everywhere, and frequently visits her children or has them visit her.

How many Katie Coopers, I often wonder, are out there? Based on my work, I believe that there are hundreds of thousands — perhaps even millions — of older Americans who are overmedicated into failing health and that we all would be a lot better off if the health care system could address the epidemic of polypharmacy.

We'd save a lot of money, too. One review,

based on seventeen studies that were published from 1976 to 1988, estimated the indirect costs of polypharmacy to be upward of $25 billion a year. And this review was conducted well before the introduction of most of the expensive "blockbuster" drugs that are in widespread use today.

One of the emotions that I must deal with on a daily basis is fear. The patients I see are often afraid of what the future holds for them and feel that they're on a downward slide healthwise. But they may fear discontinuing the medications that their doctors have prescribed. It frequently takes a lot of persuading on my part that stopping a medication — often many medications — really is the best course of action.

A study published in the *Archives of Internal Medicine* in 2010 found that there's often nothing to lose — and much to gain — from stopping many of the medications that doctors have prescribed.

"Polypharmacy itself should be conceptually perceived as 'a disease,' " the authors wrote, "with potentially more serious complications than those of the diseases these different drugs have been prescribed for."

The study documented that it's possible to withdraw medications safely and significantly from older people who are still living in the community. (The study focused on this population, as opposed to people in nursing homes or other long-term care facilities.) In fact, nearly 60 percent of the prescription medications taken by the patients in the study were able to be discontinued safely.

That, however, wasn't the most astonishing finding of the study. This, at least as I see it, was (I've added the italics):

"No significant adverse events or deaths were attributable to discontinuation, and 88 percent of patients reported global improvement in health."

In other words, nearly nine of every ten patients who stopped medications that their doctors had prescribed said that their overall health had improved as a result.

The lesson? If you think you're taking too many medications, you probably are.

Off-Limits for Older People: The Beers Criteria — A List That Could Save Your Life

Where to begin in determining whether you're using medications that might actually be harmful? If you're sixty or older — or if you're concerned about a spouse, parent, or other relative in that age group — there is, fortunately, an easy answer. It's called the Beers list.

The list was the brainchild of Mark H. Beers, MD, a widely respected geriatrician, editor in chief of the Merck Manuals, and a dear friend of mine. He was a visionary whose work has undoubtedly saved many thousands of lives a year and improved the lives of countless others in ways that we cannot possibly even imagine.

Mark's life story tells us a lot about why he did what he did. Diagnosed with type 1 diabetes when he was nine years old, Beers never allowed the disease to limit his passions or life's work. Early on, he decided that he wanted to be a doctor, but medical schools in those days summarily rejected diabetic applicants. He ended up attending the University of Vermont College of Medicine, the only school that would accept him. (Today it has a scholarship fund named after Mark.)

As a fellow in geriatrics at Harvard University in 1985, Beers saw nursing home residents routinely prescribed antipsychotic drugs like chlorpromazine (Thorazine) and thioridazine (Mellaril) to subdue them and to control the behavior of those with dementia. But Beers soon came to realize that there was no evidence of these powerful drugs' efficacy, and that many of their side effects — chief among them tardive dyskinesia, a neurological disorder characterized by repetitive, involuntary movements such as grimacing and tongue thrusting — were both horrific and irreversible. "That's where the idea for the Beers criteria was born," a former colleague, Richard W. Besdine, MD, later recalled.

The experience, I believe, impelled Beers to use his gifts as a thinker and writer to advance the field of geriatrics. I've read that his own chronic illness gave him a special empathy for older people, and I think he also saw an opportunity in geriatrics to improve the care, and the lives, of millions of old people.

He wrote the *Merck Manual of Geriatrics,* which was published in 1990 and instantly became the authoritative reference on caring for older people. The following year, he established what would soon become known as the Beers criteria — he was too self-effacing to use that term himself — through an article published in the *Archives of Internal Medicine.* This was a comprehensive list of medications that pharmacists and doctors deemed inappropriate for older people because their known risks outweighed their benefits. This "Do Not Use" list was a revolutionary idea with a revolutionary impact.

The odd fact that Beers had a very difficult time finding a medical school that would accept him never slowed him down, and I think may have put him on the path of thinking outside the box for new approaches to treating the nation's geriatric population. Anyone in the health professions who dares to challenge conventional wisdom isn't going to have an easy time of it, and I know the road that Mark traveled had more than its share of bumps.

I had the pleasure of working with him as he developed the Beers criteria and on many other committees in the American

Society of Consultant Pharmacists. Although he was a physician, Mark truly respected and welcomed input from pharmacists. We shared many ideas on how the delivery of palliative care to older people with chronic diseases was the only way to improve their lives and squeeze out every possible ounce of quality of life.

A year later, Beers became an associate editor of the Merck Manuals, where he carried on his crusade for physician and public education. In 1996 he lost his left leg below the knee to diabetes. I didn't know at the time that he was a classically trained ballet dancer, but when I later read how he kept dancing with a prosthesis after his amputation, it didn't surprise me a bit. The man was pretty much unstoppable when he put his mind to something.

He did give up dancing after he lost his other leg in 1998, but as soon as he was able to, he took up rowing in its place. He was barely past forty.

Mark Beers died in February 2009 from diabetes-related complications. I was sorry to lose a good friend — and there were so many people like me who regarded Mark as a special friend — but I was especially saddened because there is so much work yet to do in the field he pioneered.

In different years, Mark and I were each honored with the George F. Archambault Award, bestowed by the American Society of Consultant Pharmacists on someone who's had the greatest impact on the profession of pharmacy and the patients we serve. I am a pharmacist, of course, but Mark wasn't. He was the first physician ever to receive this award. And that shows, really, how much pharmacists respected Mark's hard work, professionalism, and contributions to the betterment of patient care.

I am proud to have known Mark, to have worked alongside him on some of his major projects, and just to have had the opportunity to talk with him, over lunch or just sitting around, about geriatric care. He was always an inspirational presence. While Beers's progress in improving geriatric care was cut short by diabetes, I hope that many others will step up and carry on his work and help fulfill his vision.

REQUIRED READING FOR OLDER PATIENTS — AND THEIR DOCTORS

Some prescription drugs, of course, provide real benefits to older people, but others can be lethal, either by themselves or in combination with the other medications used to treat the multiple diseases or disorders that are so often seen in this age group.

As Beers explained it some time before his death, the list is both an end point and a starting point. "Once you're taking more than two or three drugs," he said, "you have to realize that every time you add a new drug, the risk of something going wrong goes up exponentially, not linearly."

The older patients I see are often shocked to learn that they have been taking drugs — sometimes for many years — that their doctors never should have prescribed in the first place. Surely every physician who treats older patients should be familiar with the Beers criteria, but in my experience, many don't even know that such a list exists.

The patients I see frequently say, "But I've been taking this for thirty years," or something along those lines, and I'm sure they have. But now, with reduced muscle mass and impaired organ functions, the drug has become a loaded weapon with a trigger that can be pulled at any time.

When I visit nursing homes to conduct drug therapy management reviews, I see this in even starker relief. As I open chart after chart, I scan the medications on board, laboratory tests, progress notes from the nurses and physicians, and often I really cannot believe how many Beers-listed drugs

— including ones with life-threatening potential — have been prescribed. Sometimes, of course, there can be a valid reason for prescribing a drug on the Beers list to an older patient, but most often there isn't. I typically see doctors matching drugs to symptoms in knee-jerk fashion without giving much thought as to which patients might be exceptions to the prescribing rule. Older patients often are such exceptions, as the Beers criteria shows.

As alarming as it may seem, even some geriatricians are woefully ignorant about the Beers criteria. I've worked with a lot of caring and gifted geriatricians over the years, but sometimes the patients and families with whom I consult are surprised to learn that physicians can simply bill themselves as geriatricians with no special training, and often in such cases their knowledge of drug therapy management is not all that good.

This goes, too, for some of the psychiatrists who bill themselves as "board-certified geriatric psychiatrists." I've found that some of the psychiatrists who use this label mostly as a marketing device aren't all that familiar with current studies on the drugs they frequently prescribe.

Along the same lines, I'm constantly made aware of how many pharmacists, doctors, and other health care professionals don't keep current with all the changes in technology and pharmacokinetics that are constantly identifying additional problems with relatively common drugs. As a rule, these practitioners rely too heavily on information provided by pharmaceutical manufacturers and not enough on reviews that are more likely to produce unbiased results because their authors are independent of the drug companies. Their lack of skepticism about claims advanced by drug manufacturers leads to poor outcomes for patients in their care — and, in the worst cases, fatal results. Keeping up with the latest medical research in one's field takes both work and time, but it's essential to delivering the quality of care that patients deserve and should expect.

All of this is especially discouraging to me because the Beers criteria have now been around for more than twenty years. Medical professionals who ignore this approach not only endanger lives but also waste enormous amounts of money that could be put to better use in the health care system. The money that could be saved doesn't have to do just with the cost of the drugs but also with the emergency room visits, hospitalizations, extra visits to doctors and other health care providers, treatments, scans, labs, and many added costs associated with resolving the problems arising from the inappropriate use of those drugs.

Let me give you just one example of how doctors who ignore the Beers criteria multiply adverse events and send health care costs skyward. A study published in the *American Journal of Managed Care* in 2010 found that older patients who had been prescribed sedative hypnotics, which the Beers criteria classify as "high severity" drugs, were 22 percent more likely to suffer a fall or fracture than older patients in a control group who were not prescribed the drugs. In addition, the patients taking sedative hypnotics had significantly higher medical bills.

And things have gotten worse in recent years. Up until 2006, if a doctor refused to discontinue a drug in a nursing home on the recommendation of a consultant pharmacist, he or she would have to explain in writing the reason or reasons for rejecting the recommendation and why continuing the drug was medically necessary. The American Medical Association (AMA) worked long and hard to get this reversed. Fortunately, however, it failed to do so, as this would have been a huge setback for the residents of nursing homes and members of their families. Working with Sam Kidder, PharmD, the chief of the long-term care branch of the federal Health Care Financing Administration (the forerunner of the Centers for Medicare and Medicaid Services), we were able to establish a great system of checks and balances for the use of medications in older patients.

The initial victory of requiring an explanation for prescribing medication that was counter to a consultant pharmacist's recommendation had come with the passage of the 1987 Nursing Home Reform Act. This process provided extra safety for the patient. But the follow-through by the regulatory agencies was always lukewarm to none at all, because they were afraid of the repercussions that could come from a physician with enough political pull to get a surveyor fired. On the positive side, however, most physicians followed the procedure, establishing a dialogue between the clinical pharmacist and physician that furthered the best interests of the patient.

In one of the nursing homes where I do drug therapy management reviews, I run up against a geriatrician who can't stand it when I place a notation in a patient's medical records about the need for changes in medications. It infuriates the doctor so much that sometimes he sends the recommendations back in a plastic bag after he's run them through the shredder. The nursing home is between a rock and a hard place because the federal regulations clearly state, "Each resident's drug regimen must be free from unnecessary drugs." The regulations define an unnecessary drug as any drug used (1) in excessive dose, including duplicate drug therapy; (2) for excessive duration, without adequate monitoring or without adequate indications for its use; or (3) in the presence of adverse consequences indicating that the dose should be reduced or discontinued.

In my experience, nursing homes tread softly around doctors who can get them in trouble; consequently, they rarely do anything about unnecessary drugs identified by a clinical (consultant) pharmacist. All this runaround dates to 1965 and the passage of the Social Security Act, which states that the government cannot interfere with the practice of medicine. This was nearly fifty years ago, of course. But now we're in the twenty-first century and need to change outmoded ways of practicing medicine, notwithstanding the efforts of the American Medical Association to keep them in place.

Today clinical pharmacists and other

specialty health professionals have moved ahead of physicians in their knowledge of prescription drugs — and especially the use of prescription drugs in older patients. A physician, when asked to do so, should be required to explain why his or her actions on any decision are medically appropriate. This is the reason behind the 1987 Nursing Home Reform Act, as well as the regulations that the law put in place to control unnecessary and inappropriate medications in nursing homes, and, of course, the Beers criteria.

Mark Beers's original vision was to bring some sort of science to a place where no science existed, as the clinical drug trials on which we rely have historically excluded older adults. Randomized trials, which are research studies on human volunteers, have long been thought to provide the most reliable data on which drugs are effective and which aren't. He could see that older people were often prescribed the same drugs in the same doses as younger people, with little or no thought as to which medications might be inappropriate based on the vastly different pharmacodynamic and pharmacokinetic profiles of older individuals (in this case, nursing home residents).

At the heart of the Beers criteria was the idea of classifying a medication as inappropriate for older people if the potential risks associated with its use outweighed the potential benefits. He did this using something called the Delphi method, which is built around the concept of achieving consensus among a panel of experts.

Beers identified fourteen nationally recognized experts in the field and invited them to participate; all but one agreed to be part of the project. The list of medications that the thirteen-member panel developed, published in the *Archives of Internal Medicine* in 1991, focused on those widely used in nursing home settings. It quickly became known as the Beers criteria.

Beers then set about expanding the concept to all older people, not just those in institutional settings, and in 1997 an updated version of the Beers criteria was published. They were updated again in 2003, and in 2012 the American Geriatrics Society published an updated and revised version of the Beers criteria. While I have a lot of respect for this organization, I was disappointed in the 2012 list because it failed to include many newer drugs that pose manifold problems for older people.

The 2003 Beers criteria, which I generally

prefer, put drugs in two broad categories: (1) medications that should generally be avoided in persons sixty-five years or older because they are either ineffective or present unnecessarily high risks and because a safer alternative is available; and (2) medications that should not be used in older persons with specific medical conditions. The first category, in other words, is independent of the diagnosis, while the second isn't.

Here is my annotated version of the Beers criteria. I have excluded some medications because they are no longer on the market or are prescribed only rarely. Others I have organized into categories built around either the chemical structures or intended use; they are presented here first. The rest of the medications are listed in alphabetical order.

MY MEDICATIONS-TO-AVOID LIST — THE MAJOR DRUG FAMILIES

Amphetamines. Amphetamines are psychostimulant drugs of the phenethylamine class. They produce increased wakefulness and focus in association with decreased fatigue and appetite.

All amphetamines carry an FDA black-box warning and never should be prescribed to older adults, especially those with high blood pressure. (A black-box warning, so named for the black border that typically surrounds a warning on the package insert of a prescription drug, means that the drug carries a significant risk of serious or even life-threatening adverse effects. It's the strongest warning that the FDA requires.) Their adverse effects include cognitive impairment, serious mood changes, confusion, hallucinations, and abnormal heart rhythms, or cardiac arrhythmias.

I don't see amphetamine drugs prescribed all that often to geriatric patients, but I do see them. I see some amphetamine derivatives that are used to treat fatigue and the sleep disorder narcolepsy with much greater frequency. Sometimes I'll be reviewing with a family member all the drugs that a patient in a hospital or nursing home is taking. When I get to methylphenidate, which has been prescribed for narcolepsy, I explain that it's usually known by the brand name Ritalin and that it's a Schedule II controlled substance. (Drugs that are classified as Schedule II controlled substances have a currently accepted medical use but are accompanied by a high potential for abuse, which in turn may lead to severe psychological or physical dependence.) The product insert for this drug plainly warns that prescribers should proceed with caution in patients over sixty-five and that it should not be used by patients over eighty. Nonetheless, it is.

Whenever I see an elderly patient who can't sleep, is irritable, and is finding it difficult to get along in a family setting, I suspect immediately that an amphetamine or amphetamine-like drug is on board. I'll then look at the medications and see that the patient is taking one of these drugs twice a day for fatigue as well as for sleepy spells during the day and sleep apnea. At that point, it's easy to resolve his problem. If very old people aren't challenged throughout the day, they are much more likely to fall asleep, especially if they are taking drugs that can impair mobility or cause some degree of drowsiness. In these cases, we can typically change a blood pressure medication or other drug, find something for the patient to do to stay busy, and stop the stimulant use, and all those problems go away.

Antihistamines with anticholinergic properties. Antihistamines are widely used to relieve the symptoms of allergies, hay fever, and the common cold, and nearly all of them are highly anticholinergic.

Older people should not take chlorpheniramine (Chlor-Trimeton), cyproheptadine (Periactin), dexchlorpheniramine (Polaramine), diphenhydramine (Benadryl), hydroxyzine (Atarax, Vistaril), oxybutynin (Ditropan), or tolterodine (Detrol). Like other anticholinergic drugs, all can cause a wide variety of adverse effects, including constipation, difficulty urinating, blurred vision, confusion, and short-term memory problems.

Talk about a pharmaceutical Pandora's box.

A man from California called me recently because his doctor had him taking finasteride (Proscar) to treat his enlarged prostate and then put him on extended-release Detrol LA to keep him from having to get up so many times during the night to go to the bathroom. With his wife on the other line, the man complained that he hallucinates all night, can't sleep, and can't go to the bathroom at all.

This is another case of a doctor ignoring, or not even being aware of, the Beers criteria, to the patient's detriment. Using any anticholinergic drug in a patient with an enlarged prostate, or benign prostatic hyperplasia (BPH), will restrict his urine flow and cause serious problems that may lead to a trip to the emergency room, serious urinary infections, or both. I advised him to call the doctor the next day and tell him that he was stopping the Detrol LA, and why.

Why would a physician prescribe the antihistamine meclizine (Antivert) to an eighty-year-old for dizziness? What does he think this anticholinergic drug will do to help the dizziness, when the drug causes it in every case? Why would a physician prescribe Periactin to an eighty-three-year-old as an appetite stimulant, when it will cause many more problems than being a few pounds underweight ever could? Why would a physician prescribe Vistaril or Atarax to a seventy-five-year-old for anxiety, when the confusion and hallucinations will exacerbate anxiety in almost every patient? And if you think I'm saying all this just to scare you, I am. If you have glaucoma and take these drugs, you can go *blind!*

Antihistamines with lower anticholinergic profiles, such as loratadine (Claritin) and cetirizine (Zyrtec), are better choices for older adults, preferably at reduced doses.

Antipsychotic (neuroleptic) drugs. This family of drugs includes chlorpromazine (Thorazine), haloperidol (Haldol), mesoridazine (Serentil), olanzapine (Zyprexa), quetiapine (Seroquel), risperidone (Risperdal), thioridazine (Mellaril), thiothixene (Navane), and ziprasidone (Geodon), as well as perphenazine-amitriptyline (Triavil), a drug (see page 155) that combines an antipsychotic with a tricyclic antidepressant. These are all medications with powerful tranquilizing properties that are used to treat the symptoms of schizophrenia and other serious psychotic mental disorders, especially those that involve hallucinations and delusions.

As a starting point, it's important to remember that only 0.1 percent of people sixty-five and older — or one in every one thousand — are diagnosed as having active schizophrenia, which is by far the most common serious psychotic mental disorder. Yet prescriptions for these powerful drugs continue to be written in alarming numbers, decades after their dangers were first documented.

More than twenty years ago, in a study published in the *Journal of the American Medical Association,* lead author Mark Beers wrote, "The usefulness of antipsychotic medications in nonpsychotic, elderly patients has been questioned . . . The high frequency of toxic reactions to these drugs is well documented, with many older patients who take them experiencing ortho-static hypotension, Parkinson's syndrome, tardive dyskinesia [a neuromuscular disorder characterized by repetitive, involuntary movements, such as grimacing and tongue thrusting], akathisia [a subjective feeling of restlessness and the urge to move about], worsened confusion, constipation, oversedation, and urinary incontinence."

These sometimes horrific side effects, in fact, were largely the impetus for the 1987 Nursing Home Reform Act and the regulations that seek to limit the use of psychotropic, or mind-altering, medications, particularly antipsychotics, in long-term care facilities.

Although antipsychotic drugs are not approved for use in the treatment of Alzheimer's disease or any type of dementia, they are often prescribed for that purpose. They are also prescribed, studies show, for an alarming number of nonpsychiatric disorders. In the nation's nursing homes, where antipsychotics have been used improperly to sedate residents or to control nonpsychotic behaviors, these drugs have been the leading cause of adverse drug reactions.

These include powerful sedative effects (up to twenty-four hours of drug-induced sleep after a single dose), a wide array of anticholinergic effects (dry mouth, urine retention, confusion, and so on), extrapyramidal symptoms (antipsychotics may cause tardive dyskinesia in as many as 40 percent of the people over the age of sixty who take them, for example), and lowering blood pressure to dangerous levels. Antipsychotics are thought to be the leading cause of drug-induced hip fractures. The list of problems really just goes on and on and on, and includes heart failure and sudden death.

Most of the patients on antipsychotics I see in my office and in the nursing homes where I do drug therapy management reviews never should have been put on them in the first place. Often the symptoms that lead a doctor to prescribe the antipsychotic — confusion, delirium, or hallucinations, for example — are being caused by other drugs, including antibiotics, antihistamines, antidepressants, sedatives, and steroids, to name just a few.

All antipsychotics now carry an FDA black-box warning that they can increase the risk of death in patients with dementia because of heart attacks or pneumonia. Nonetheless, a study released in 2011 found that about one in seven nursing home residents age sixty-five or older had been prescribed new-generation antipsychotics, notwithstanding the black-box warning, in the six-month period studied.

In 2009 the pharmaceutical giant Eli Lilly and Company pleaded guilty to illegally marketing Zyprexa as a treatment for elderly patients with dementia and paid $1.4 billion in criminal penalties and settlements in four civil lawsuits. Its blockbuster antipsychotic had US sales of nearly $3 billion in 2010.

But an investigation published last year by ProPublica, a nonprofit organization that's won two Pulitzer Prizes for reporting, found that a doctor named as a codefendant in one of the civil lawsuits — for allegedly taking kickbacks to prescribe the drug extensively at more than one hundred nursing homes in Florida — never was pursued.

What's the truth? We may never know.

Barbiturates. Because they act as central nervous system depressants, barbiturates produce a wide spectrum of effects, from mild sedation to total anesthesia. They are also used as anxiolytics (antianxiety agents), hypnotics, and anticonvulsants (to treat epileptic seizures, for example).

Barbiturates can produce many unpredictable responses in older adults, who typically are more sensitive to their sedative effects but also highly susceptible to such adverse effects as confusion, agitation, delirium, hyperactivity, and other cognitive changes.

I see quite a few very old patients with epilepsy who still need a barbiturate — typically, phenobarbital in combination with phenytoin (Dilantin), an anticonvulsant — to prevent seizures. In these cases, stopping or tapering off the barbiturate is almost impossible because the patient's body has been accustomed to this chemistry for so long.

Older patients sometimes develop tremors that aren't associated with an underlying medical problem (such as Parkinson's disease) and don't point to a serious medical condition. These "essential tremors," sometimes referred to as senile tremors, affect an estimated four million Americans, most of them older than fifty. Doctors often prescribe the anticonvulsant primidone (Mysoline) for essential tremors, but this drug actually metabolizes to phenobarbital, with all its attendant adverse effects. Many other medications are available that treat essential tremors more safely and effectively.

Benzodiazepines. Benzodiazepines are typically used to treat insomnia, anxiety, and panic disorders.

Because they are metabolized in the liver, and because the liver stops making some of the isozymes that metabolize drugs as you grow older, benzodiazepines can accumulate at dangerous levels in the bodies of older adults. Long-acting benzodiazepines, which are cleared out of the body more slowly, are thus the most dangerous. The Beers criteria include six long-acting benzodiazepines — chlordiazepoxide (Librium, Mitran), clorazepate (Tranxene), diazepam (Valium), flurazepam (Dalmane), quazepam (Doral, Dormalin), and temazepam (Restoril) — as well as the short-acting benzodiazepines alprazolam (Xanax), estazolam (ProSom), lorazepam (Ativan), oxazepam (Serax), and triazolam (Halcion).

The benzodiazepine drugs can cause unsteadiness, dizziness, and even vertigo, increasing the risk of falls and fractures. Studies show that older people taking benzodiazepines see their risk of falls rise by as much as 70 percent and their risk of hip fracture by at least 50 percent. This is all the more alarming because these drugs have no proven long-term benefits and are often prescribed unnecessarily.

Additionally, some of the benzodiazepine drugs — typically, the ones labeled as hypnotics — stay in the body so long that the residual sedation can lead to problems with driving or working with machinery. There is some evidence, too, that long-term use of benzodiazepines can lead to cognitive impairments.

This class of drugs is so inappropriately used in older patients across the board that often a primary reason for a patient's admission to a nursing home is the past use of these drugs. Broken arms, hips, legs and other adverse events that require surgery and then a long recovery could have been avoided if the physician had merely delved deeper into the patient's sleep problems before prescribing a hypnotic sleeping pill. Was another drug on board interfering with the patient's ability to sleep? Was the patient experiencing too much anxiety or stress for some reason? Was pain or some other organic problem causing or contributing to the patient's sleep disorder? Answering those questions might have precluded the need for the hypnotic and, ultimately, allowed the patient to continue to live independently at home.

Some time ago, an eighty-six-year-old woman was referred to me for an evaluation after she drove her car through the back wall of her garage. Her daughter believed that she was too old to drive and needed to live in a nursing home. "She can't even live on her own at home anymore," the daughter told me, "and this accident proves that she can't drive, either."

Well, it didn't take long for me to discover the problem. The woman scored a perfect 30 out of 30 on the Mini-Mental State Examination (MMSE), a questionnaire-type test that's used to screen for cognitive impairment, but a look at the drugs she was taking showed four different benzodiazepines prescribed for her to take at different times of the day. She had driven through the back of her garage because she'd fallen asleep! We removed all the rogue drugs and a few more, and now she is driving once again, volunteering as a Pink Lady at the local hospital, and living independently in her own house. How different this all would have been if the woman's physician had even the most basic familiarity with the Beers criteria.

Estrogens (Premarin, Climara, Cenestin). Estrogen, a hormone, is used to treat hot flashes in menopausal women. Some brands of estrogen are also used to treat vaginal dryness, itching, or burning. Estrogen has also been promoted as having long-term benefits, preventing heart disease and osteoporosis.

Most of the claims for estrogen therapy have been disproved. In fact, estrogens must now carry FDA black-box warnings that they increase the risk of endometrial (uterine) cancer, breast cancer, cardiovascular disease, and dementia. Additionally, the claims for bone enhancement are questionable, and estrogens are no longer approved by the FDA for the treatment of osteoporosis. In 2002 a large, long-term clinical trial of estrogen therapy in postmenopausal women sponsored by the National Institutes of Health had to be stopped three years earlier than scheduled because of increases in such serious adverse events such as heart attack, stroke, and some forms of cancer.

With all the information available about the dangers of hormone replacement therapy (HRT), I often wonder why any doctor would prescribe estrogen to a female patient.

Some time ago, a sixty-eight-year-old woman came to see me, accompanied by her husband. She had been diagnosed with bipolar disorder (formerly known as manic-depressive disorder) years back and was taking so much lamotrigine (Lamictal), bupropion (Wellbutrin), and mirtazapine

(Remeron) — all antidepressants, all prescribed by one psychiatrist — that she couldn't carry on a conversation without getting sidetracked. Her husband had come with her both to explain the problems she was having and to help her understand what I was telling her.

As I perused the list of medications that the woman was taking, I saw several different forms of estrogen therapy as well. The amount of diuretics was high, consistent with excessive estrogen therapy, and the risk of a fatal stroke was high, consistent with inadequate treatment for chronic high blood pressure, or hypertension. We slowly tapered off the estrogen therapy over sixty days or so before we proceeded to challenge the assumption of bipolar disorder. My thinking was that if we could stop some of the hormonal brain chemistry, which is known to produce wide mood swings and abnormal behavior, we could possibly eliminate the heavy-duty psychotropic drugs.

Today she is taking diltiazem CD for her blood pressure, a low dose of torsemide (Demadex) for edema, omega-3 fish oil supplements and aspirin for stroke prevention, and venlafaxine (Effexor XR) for anxiety and depression, which also helps with her sleeping. To reach our therapeutic goals, we had to slowly titrate out all the psychotropic drugs, a process that took about four months. She is happy, shows no signs of any bipolar disorder, and travels with her husband — they are both retired — everywhere. In this case, as in so many others, the doctors treating her seemed to have no knowledge of the Beers criteria — and next to no common sense.

Nonsteroidal anti-inflammatory drugs (NSAIDs). This family of drugs includes indomethacin (Indocin, Indocin SR), ibuprofen (Motrin, Advil, Medipren), naproxen (Aleve, Anaprox, Midol Extended Relief), meloxicam (Mobic), ketorolac (Toradol), piroxicam (Feldene), and oxaprozin (Daypro). NSAIDs are used to relieve moderate to severe pain, tenderness, swelling, and stiffness caused by osteoarthritis, rheumatoid arthritis, and ankylosing spondylitis (severe arthritis that affects mainly the spine). They are also used to treat shoulder pain caused by bursitis (inflammation of fluid-filled sacs that protect the joints from stress) and tendinitis (inflammation or irritation of a tendon) and to treat acute gouty arthritis (attacks of severe joint pain and swelling caused by a buildup of certain substances in the joints).

NSAIDs surely serve a purpose, but they are not at all friendly to older people, who are more likely to have reduced liver and kidney function. All NSAIDs can cause gastrointestinal bleeding that may lead to hospitalization or death. The larger the dose or the longer you take them, the greater your risk.

Often an older patient will take an NSAID at bedtime each night to relieve joint and muscle pain, start bleeding internally without any warning or symptom, and bleed to death.

Although NSAIDs can vary in their degree of gastrointestinal toxicity, there is no reason for older adults to use them when so many other, safer analgesic drugs are available. I believe strongly that this class of drugs should not be sold over the counter. There are so many different patient conditions and chemistry problems that need to be considered before they are used that making NSAIDs available in nonprescription form does a real disservice, and poses real dangers, to the people who buy them. A patient who takes four Advil at bedtime for sleep is at risk for a serious and potentially fatal GI bleed at any time.

MY MEDICATIONS-TO-AVOID LIST

Amiodarone (Cordarone). Amiodarone is used to treat and prevent certain types of life-threatening arrythmias (irregular heartbeats), especially ventricular arrhythmias.

In my judgment, it is a last-resort antiarrhythmic drug. Amiodarone can cause toxic reactions in the liver, lungs, thyroid gland, and heart, and more than 80 percent of those who take the drug experience adverse, sometimes fatal, effects. The most dangerous of these is pulmonary fibrosis, in which lung tissue becomes damaged and scarred. Amiodarone is so dangerous, in fact, that it carries an FDA black-box warning that the drug "has several potentially fatal toxicities."

A newer relative of this drug, dronedarone (Multaq), is also used to treat arrhythmias, but its side effects profile isn't any better. It too carries an FDA black-box warning.

Amiodarone may be needed for a very short time in the hospital setting to reregulate the heart, but its use should stop at the hospital door when the patient leaves. It wreaks all kinds of havoc on the thyroid system, which controls how quickly the body uses energy, makes proteins, and reacts to other hormones.

I see patients both in nursing homes and in my office who have been diagnosed with chronic obstructive pulmonary disease (COPD) — chronic bronchitis or emphysema, or both — and are on every bronchodilator (medications used to relax and expand the bronchial airways, making it easier to breathe) known to mankind. Some are on oxygen too. Then I look at the drugs that have been prescribed and see that the patient has been on amiodarone for the past year and a half. At this point, I know that the patient doesn't have COPD; he or she has drug-induced pulmonary fibrosis, and the disease is in the final stages. Tragically, nothing can be done at this point, and the pulmonary fibrosis will continue to smother the patient to death. It's a ghastly disease that could have been totally avoided. What was the physician thinking when he or she started the patient on this dangerous drug?

Amitriptyline (Elavil). Amitriptyline, a tricyclic antidepressant, is used to treat symptoms of depression.

This drug is so highly anticholinergic that it should always be ruled out in older patients. Its adverse effects, as with all anticholinergic drugs, include constipation, difficulty urinating, blurred vision, confusion and short-term memory problems, and even cardiac arrhythmias.

Amitriptyline is sometimes prescribed as an analgesic for neuropathic pain, which is logical because this type of pain arises from the body's nervous systems. (It works, however, in only about a third of the patients who take it for this purpose.) This is another instance where I often hear something along the lines of, "But I've been taking it for thirty years without any problems." Well, I have to explain, you were just forty years old then, and now you are seventy, and the drug is making your cardiac problems worse. Years ago, the patient should have been switched to a drug that would relieve the pain without causing all the problems that come with amitriptyline.

Belladonna alkaloids and phenobarbital (Donnatal). Donnatal is a combination of three belladonna alkaloids, which are antispasmodic drugs, with phenobarbital, a barbiturate. (See page 115.) It is used to relieve cramping pains in conditions such as irritable bowel syndrome and spastic colon. It is also used with other medicines to treat ulcers. It is highly anticholinergic.

With the introduction of H_2 blockers

(cimetidine and ranitidine, for example) and proton pump inhibitors, the belladonna alkaloids — atropine, hyoscyamine, dicyclomine, and scopolamine — lost their standing in the treatment of gastrointestinal disorders. Like other highly anticholinergic drugs, they can cause constipation, difficulty urinating, blurred vision, confusion and short-term memory problems, and problems with many other involuntary body processes.

These are just some of the anticholinergic side effects of belladonna alkaloids. But this drug also contains phenobarbital, which compounds many of these adverse effects and exacerbates cognition problems.

The issue with stopping Donnatal is that patients have to be tapered off the drug very slowly. Rebound acid hypersecretion (elevated gastric acid brought on as the drug is withdrawn) is a big problem, and combined with the psychological and physiological dependence brought on by the phenobarbital, we're always in for a bumpy ride in removing the drug. If successful, though, typically patients are amazed at how many of the problems that have inched up on them over the years of taking this drug vanish.

The FDA has concluded that there is no

evidence that Donnatal is effective for any indication, which is sufficient reason not to take it. In my opinion, it should have been removed from the market long ago.

Bisacodyl (Dulcolax). Bisacodyl, a stimulant laxative, is used to treat constipation. It also is used to empty the bowels before surgery and examinations such as X-ray procedures using barium enemas.

You never should take bisacodyl or another stimulant laxative routinely for simple constipation. Chronic use of the drug gradually robs your large intestine of its ability to work efficiently and can lead to electrolyte loss, vitamin and mineral deficiencies, and serious bowel dysfunctions such as cathartic colon, a disease of the large intestine. Long-term use of bisacodyl can also cause hypokalemia, an abnormally low level of potassium in the blood, which can lead to dangerous arrhythmias, kidney damage, and paralysis.

One of the big problems is that many older people grew up taking mineral oil, castor oil, Fletcher's Castoria, Carter's Little Liver Pills (now sold as Carter's Little Pills), Phillips' Milk of Magnesia, or one of the many similar products to "stay regular," as the saying goes. Many people believe that staying regular means having one bowel movement a day, but that's not true for everyone. The general range of *regular,* in fact, is from three times a day to three times a week. But just try convincing the average eighty-year-old of that, and you've got a battle on your hands. Getting the patient to switch to mild bulk laxatives or stool softeners often takes some time, since "Mama took castor oil every Friday night to stay regular."

Carisoprodol (Soma). Carisoprodol, a muscle relaxant, is used to relieve pain and discomfort caused by strains, sprains, and other muscle injuries. Carisoprodol is broken down in the body to meprobamate (see page 151), a Schedule IV controlled substance.

Carisoprodol's anticholinergic properties make it inappropriate for older people; the same goes for its sedative effects. The drug can cause drowsiness, dizziness, confusion, slowed thinking, loss of balance and coordination, fainting, and insomnia, as well as many, many other adverse effects.

The paramount problem with using carisoprodol long term is psychological dependence. The manufacturer warns that Soma never should be used for more than two to three weeks to treat acute musculoskeletal discomfort. That's the point, in my experience, at which the confusion, hallucinations, and cognition problems dominate, and the patient's family brings him or her to see me.

It's very difficult to taper any patient off of Soma, let alone a sixty-, seventy-, or eighty-year-old. But if the older patient is ever to experience better cognition and independence, it must be done.

Cascara sagrada. Cascara sagrada, a stimulant laxative made from a species of buckthorn, is used to treat constipation or before rectal or bowel examinations or surgery.

This is an old drug that has been around since 1939. In 1996 the FDA classified cascara sagrada as a Category III laxative (meaning that additional data are needed to establish its safety). Six years later, the FDA changed the classification to Category II, thus banning its use in over-the-counter laxative products.

You never should take cascara sagrada or any other stimulant laxative on a routine basis for simple constipation. Chronic use can lead to electrolyte imbalance, weakness, fainting, stomach pain, and urine discoloration.

■ ■ ■ ■

Chlorpropamide (Diabinese). Chlorpropamide, a sulfonylurea drug, is used — sometimes with other medications — to treat type 2 diabetes, a condition in which the body either fails to make enough insulin to control the amount of sugar in the blood or is unable to properly use the insulin that it does produce.

Because chlorpropamide has a very long half-life (sixty hours or longer), it can cause profound hypoglycemia (low blood sugar), leading to falls; hyponatremia (an abnormally low level of sodium in the blood); and SIADH (syndrome of inappropriate antidiuretic hormone secretion), a condition caused by abnormally low sodium levels in the body. In patients with impaired renal function, the adverse events are much higher.

Finally, the package insert for Diabinese notes that its safety and effectiveness in patients sixty-five and older "has not been properly evaluated in clinical studies."

We've made so much progress in understanding type 2 diabetes and treating the disease in older patients that there really is no need for Diabinese and other sulfonylurea drugs. The type 2 diabetic usually makes enough insulin, but the receptor sites on all the body's cells are unable to take it in. The newer-generation drugs work by stimulating the receptor sites to use the body's own insulin.

For many patients on sulfonylurea therapy, the problems begin first thing in the morning. Let's say that a patient gets up in the morning to eat breakfast, takes his sulfonylurea medicine, and reads the newspaper for a while. He then takes a shower, falls in the bathtub, and breaks his arm. In taking the old-generation sulfonylurea drug, he's allowed his blood sugar level to peak and then gone into hypoglycemia in the shower and passed out. The hypoglycemia-induced problems of severe fatigue and syncope (loss of consciousness) are common in every older patient who takes a sulfonylurea drug.

Chlorzoxazone (Paraflex, Parafon Forte DCS). Chlorzoxazone is used to relieve pain and stiffness caused by muscle strains and sprains.

Because of its sedative effects, chlorzoxazone falls into the do-not-use category for older people, and it also can cause irreversible and sometimes fatal liver toxicity.

This drug, a central nervous system

(CNS) suppressant, can cause headaches, depression, amnesia, and, in older patients with impaired liver function, irreversible liver disease that can be fatal. Whenever I see chlorzoxazone being used, it tells me right off the bat that the patient's physician doesn't understand the drug and how it works and, in all likelihood, is totally unfamiliar with the Beers criteria.

Cimetidine (Tagamet). Cimetidine, an H_2 blocker, is used to treat ulcers, gastroesophageal reflux disease (GERD), and conditions where the stomach produces too much acid, such as Zollinger-Ellison syndrome. Cimetidine is available in nonprescription strengths, and in those forms is typically used to prevent and treat the symptoms of heartburn associated with acid indigestion and sour stomach.

Cimetidine was the first of the H_2 blockers. In older people, it can cause dizziness, confusion, and hallucinations. Because it works by literally shutting down the liver, it interferes with the body's ability to metabolize other drugs and can cause acute liver injury.

Back in 1976, when Tagamet was introduced (before the Beers criteria were published), it was considered a miracle drug for stomach disorders. At the time, I had an eighty-one-year-old nursing home patient who was on 10 milligrams of the tranquilizer chlordiazepoxide (Librium) three times a day for agitation and who had recently been prescribed Tagamet because she complained of stomach pain.

The Librium, a benzodiazepine, was wholly inappropriate, and the Tagamet, by shutting down the patient's liver, was causing the Librium to linger in her body for days. This induced a coma, and everyone thought the woman was dying.

From the beginning, I had believed that Tagamet's hepatic shutdown would prevent any liver-metabolized drugs from clearing the patient's body and present very serious hazards. So I wrote up my suggestion to the physician to stop both drugs, saying that I believed the patient would then wake up from the coma.

The doctor refused and responded that he had been practicing medicine for thirty years, knew all about the drugs he prescribed, and didn't need any help from me.

A little while after that, a nurse told me the rest of the story. The physician had gone back to his office and called his contact at Smith Kline & French, Tagamet's manufacturer, to tell him about the "foolish pharmacist" who was spreading misinformation about its drug. Lo and behold, however, the company representative asked the doctor to find out where I had obtained my research.

As it turned out, Smith Kline & French (now GlaxoSmithKline) was preparing to warn physicians that this was a serious adverse event associated with Tagamet, and the doctor's contact apparently told him that he had a very smart consultant pharmacist helping him. The physician never acknowledged this to me, but he reversed course and accepted my advice. The patient woke up from her coma (and lived for five more years), and from that moment on, I didn't have to worry about that doctor rejecting any more of my recommendations. While I do credit Tagamet with opening the door to vast improvements in the H_2 blockers that have helped many patients avoid stomach ulcer surgery, I believe that the drug is too potent to be sold over the counter and is a definite no-no for older patients, just as the 2003 Beers criteria suggest.

Clonidine (Catapres). Clonidine, an alpha-agonist hypotensive agent, is used alone or in combination with other medications to treat high blood pressure.

Because clonidine is excreted largely by the kidneys, the greater the degree of renal impairment in a patient, the higher the concentration of the drug. The buildup of clonidine in the body will cause dizziness, loss of glucose control, loss of consciousness, and cognitive problems.

I see this all the time in patients. Because older people have less lean body mass and hence less renal function than younger people, you can always expect problems when using a drug that is cleared primarily through the kidneys.

Many of the drugs used to treat benign prostatic hyperplasia (BPH) are also alpha-blockers, a class of blood pressure medications that stop the hormone norepinephrine from constricting small arteries and veins, thereby improving blood flow. I'll see a patient on a twice-daily dose of Catapres or a Catapres Patch (which delivers the drug continuously) and on Flomax to treat his BPH, and he complains that every time he bends over to tie his shoes or pick up something on the floor, he blacks out. Or he stands up from a sitting position and just falls over. The problem is that he's overloaded on alpha-blockers and experiencing serious orthostatic hypotension. This means that the blood pressure to the brain is low,

so that when he makes any abrupt movements, the blood essentially leaves the brain,
causing him to black out. This, of course,
leads frequently to falls and bone fractures.

Cyclobenzaprine (Flexeril). Cyclobenzaprine, a muscle relaxant, is used to relieve
pain and discomfort caused by strains,
sprains, and other muscle injuries.

Flexeril's anticholinergic and sedative effects make it inappropriate for older people,
and the frequency and severity of adverse
events associated with its use are greatest in
people over sixty — and cause the greatest
morbidity in this age group.

Not long ago, an old gentleman called me
at six o'clock in the morning from the
sheriff's office, where he was being held for
attacking his wife after accusing her of steal-
ing his money and having an affair with a
neighbor. His doctor wanted to have him
committed to a psychiatric hospital for
observation and evaluation.

It didn't take much detective work for me
to figure out what had happened. The day
before the episode, the man had gone to his
physician's office complaining of a crick in
his neck and left with a prescription for
Flexeril. He'd filled the prescription right
away, taken a pill at bedtime, and become

disoriented almost instantly. He began hallucinating, became violent with his wife, and called the sheriff's office to come get her for all her wrongdoings. Well, they got him instead. When I explained everything to the officer and assured him that this was an adverse event from a prescription drug, the man was released and allowed to return home. At that point, I asked his doctor to prescribe tramadol (Ultram) for his neck pain and to forget about using Flexeril in an older patient ever again. When I mentioned the Beers criteria to the physician, it was clear to me that he had no idea what I meant.

Desiccated thyroid (Armour Thyroid). Desiccated (dried) thyroid extract products are used to control the symptoms of hypothyroidism, in a condition in which the thyroid gland doesn't make enough thyroid hormone. This product, which the FDA approved in 1939, is derived from the thyroid gland of a pig.

Numerous studies have found the synthetic thyroid hormone levothyroxine (Levoxyl, Synthroid) to be the preferred treatment for hypothyroidism. There are wide variations in two of the thyroid hormones — levothyroxine (T4) and liothyronine (T3) — in desiccated thyroid extract, which can make continuous therapy extremely difficult. Because the hormonal content of levothyroxine is standardized, the effects of the drug are more predictable. Changing to levothyroxine should be done slowly, with thyroid-stimulating hormone (TSH) levels checked every fourteen days until the appropriate dosage is determined. (TSH is excreted by the pituitary gland, causing the thyroid gland to make the hormones T3 and T4, which help control metabolism.)

Dicyclomine (Bentyl). Dicyclomine, an antispasmodic drug, is used to relieve cramping pains in conditions such as irritable bowel syndrome and spastic colon. It is also used, with other medicines, to treat ulcers. It is highly anticholinergic.

Older people who take dicyclomine at the effective adult dose of 160 milligrams per day experience unacceptably high rates of adverse effects. Like other highly anticholinergic drugs, dicyclomine can cause constipation, difficulty urinating, blurred vision, confusion and short-term memory problems, and problems with many other involuntary processes of the body.

If you have glaucoma, blindness is a very

high risk. In older patients, many of the indications for this drug bring about adverse events. A sixty-seven-year-old man recently came to see me with multiple gastrointestinal problems: GI reflux, serious stomach pain, nausea, bloody vomit, and constant diarrhea. He was taking meloxicam for arthritis, a proton pump inhibitor (PPI) for acid reflux, an H_2 blocker for heartburn, sucralfate (Carafate) for ulcers, and dicyclomine (Bentyl) for the irritable bowel syndrome. The doctor had also put him on iron supplements to improve his blood count and a host of antidiarrhea drugs.

With all these drugs on board, it was no surprise that he had so many complaints. The topper of this pharmaceutical spree was the meloxicam, a nonsteroidal anti-inflammatory drug that never should be used in older adults and causes multiple gastrointestinal problems, including ulcers, perforated ulcers, gastric pain, and eventual GI bleeds and death. The blood loss was already present, and the iron supplements were of no benefit because the PPI and H_2 blocker were keeping his stomach at a basic pH and not allowing the iron to break down and be absorbed. First we stopped the meloxicam, then slowly tapered away the PPI, then stopped the H_2 blocker, and then the dicyclomine. I didn't believe that he had irritable bowel syndrome, and, as it turned out, he didn't.

He was left with an H_2 blocker on an as-needed basis for heartburn plus tramadol with acetaminophen (Tylenol) for any arthritic pain or general pain. All his original symptoms subsided.

Dipyridamole (Persantine). Dipyridamole is used with other drugs to reduce the risk of blood clots after heart valve replacement surgery. A combination of extended-release dipyridamole and aspirin is marketed under the brand name Aggrenox.

Studies have shown that dipyridamole can accumulate at unacceptably high concentrations in the blood of people over sixty-five. This puts them at a very high risk of orthostatic hypotension, which can lead to fainting and falling.

This drug was around in the late 1960s for treating angina through its action as a vasodilator — a medication that opens blood vessels. It proved to be problematic then, and its use faded until about 1986, when it was approved as a platelet inhibitor based on questionable and controversial studies that were suggestive rather than conclusive.

No matter the dose in the older patient, dipyridamole caused serious problems with vertigo and orthostatic hypotension, just as it had in the past, and the drug once again fell out of favor. Sometime later a pharmaceutical company combined 200 milligrams of dipyridamole with 25 milligrams of aspirin and marketed the resulting product, Aggrenox, as being twice as effective as aspirin alone in preventing the formation of blood clots. The Antiplatelet Trialists' Collaboration, a team of more than fifty independent researchers, had concluded in 1988, after reviewing all available randomized trials, that this combination was no more effective in stroke reduction than aspirin alone and that dipyridamole had no role in the treatment of thromboembolic disorders, in which blood clots threaten to block blood vessels.

A few years back, a retired high school coach made an appointment with me to discuss his health problems and medicines. At seventy-nine, he had some major cardiac problems, but he was still active and liked to play golf three times a week. He was experiencing some serious difficulties on the greens, however, as he'd become extremely dizzy whenever he leaned down to line up a putt.

I noticed right away that he was taking Aggrenox twice a day. I explained to him that this drug was no better than a full-strength aspirin (325 milligrams) alone and that the dipyridamole was causing his dizzy spells on the golf course. He said that his neurologist had prescribed the dipyridamole and talked very favorably about its benefits. In my written report, I recommended stopping the dipyridamole-aspirin combination and relying instead on a full-strength aspirin daily.

A few days later, the man called me back to tell me that his neurologist was very angry with him, saying that he had a lot of training and asking if the man was going to take the word of a pharmacist over his opinion. I told the coach that I would send him a copy of a letter that the Food and Drug Administration had sent to the manufacturer demanding that it contact all physicians and correct the false information about the drug's efficacy that it had previously presented to them. He gave the letter to his neurologist, which only inflamed the situation, and he was told that if he didn't trust him to find another neurologist. The patient stopped the combination drug on his own and started taking an enteric-coated full-strength aspirin every day. As his dizziness went away, his golf game improved, leaving him happy indeed. (Enteric coatings prevent the release of medication before it reaches the small intestine.)

I find that most specialists — like this patient's neurologist — aren't familiar with the Beers criteria, possibly because they generally don't treat older patients or follow up on the drug outcomes.

Disopyramide (Norpace, Norpace CR). Disopyramide is used to treat arrhythmias.

The drug is similar to procainamide (Pronestyl, Procan-SR, Procanbid) and quinidine (Quinidex) in its pharmacologic action, but its significant anticholinergic properties make it inappropriate for older people. Like other anticholinergic drugs, disopyramide can cause a wide variety of adverse effects, including constipation, difficulty urinating, blurred vision, and confusion and short-term memory problems. It can also cause congestive heart failure in older adults.

The FDA black-box warning for disopyramide states that "the use of Norpace or Norpace CR as well as other antiarrhythmic agents should be reserved for patients with life-threatening ventricular arrhythmias," and goes on to note its "excessive mortality" rate compared with other drugs used to treat these conditions.

Doxazosin (Cardura, Cardura XL). Doxazosin, an alpha-blocker, is used in men to treat the symptoms of an enlarged prostate. It is also used alone or in combination with other medications to treat high blood pressure.

This mild antihypertensive drug has been found to shrink the prostate gland. However, like all alpha-blockers, it puts older adults at an unacceptably high risk for orthostatic hypotension, which can lead to fainting and falling.

Many people assume that adverse events are rare, but in my experience, nearly every man who takes doxazosin will experience orthostatic hypotension. Occasionally a physician will double the dose when the prostate doesn't respond, and this only exacerbates the problem.

Benign prostatic hyperplasia (BPH) is a very difficult condition to treat. Because of the problems with the orthostatic hypotension, I do not recommend the use of alpha-blockers, because at some point the patient is going to have a serious fall. The best way to treat this problem is with surgery. A surgical procedure known as TURP (transurethral resection of the prostate), in which part of the prostate gland is removed, or a newer microwave-reduction procedure known as TUMT (transurethral microwave therapy) can cure the problem for twenty or more years without the adverse effects posed by many of the drugs used to treat BPH.

Ergoloid mesylates (Hydergine). This drug, first marketed in the United States in 1953, has long been used to treat dementia and age-related cognitive impairment (such as in Alzheimer's disease), as well as in the convalescent period after a stroke. Its actual mechanism of action is not known.

Benefits from the use of this drug are difficult if not impossible to find. A study published in the *New England Journal of Medicine* in 1990 found ergoloid mesylates to be totally ineffective for mild to moderate Alzheimer's, and to actually accelerate patients' mental decline, while an article in the *Journal of the American Medical Association* the following year noted that this treatment "has been convincingly demonstrated to be of no value."

Ethacrynic acid (Edecrin). Ethacrynic acid, a so-called water pill, is used to treat fluid retention caused by various medical problems. It is a potent loop diuretic used in the management of edema (the abnormal accumulation of fluid beneath the skin or in one or more cavities of the body) associated with various causes, including congestive heart failure, cirrhosis of the liver, and kidney disease.

Ethacrynic acid is associated with a high incidence of ototoxicity (ear damage that leads to hearing loss), making it inappropriate in older adults. In my judgment, torsemide (Demadex) is the loop diuretic of choice in treating older patients.

Ferrous sulfate (iron). Ferrous sulfate is used to treat or prevent iron-deficiency anemia, a type of anemia caused by insufficient iron.

The problems with using it in older patients are almost entirely dose related; dosing in this population should never exceed 325 milligrams a day. This medication is broken down in the gut and absorbed in the small intestine. Because only about 10 percent of ferrous sulfate is absorbed, the use of other medications — H_2 blockers, proton pump inhibitors, and antacids, for example — will inhibit absorption, as will food. Increasing the dose of ferrous sulfate above 325 milligrams a day only exacerbates the problems of constipation, nausea, and an inflamed esophagus (esophagitis), as well as anorexia.

Before your doctor starts you on this drug, he or she should order a ferritin-level blood test to confirm that you actually have iron-deficiency anemia. Abnormally low levels of ferritin, a protein in the body that binds to iron, may point to anemia brought about by insufficient iron in the blood.

Fluoxetine (Prozac). Fluoxetine, a selective serotonin reuptake inhibitor (SSRI), is used to treat depression, obsessive-compulsive disorder, some eating disorders, and panic attacks. It was the first SSRI on the market.

Fluoxetine is an inappropriate antidepressant for older adults for a variety of reasons. For one thing, many older people lack certain liver enzymes that are needed for the drug to be effective. This drug can also cause the sodium level in the blood to drop (a condition known as hyponatremia), which, in turn, can cause symptoms such as drowsiness, confusion, muscle twitching, and convulsions. Older people are especially susceptible to this adverse effect. The use of fluoxetine can also lead to anorexia and insomnia.

Finally, a major study published in the *British Medical Journal* in 2011 found that SSRIs may not be as safe for older adults as other antidepressants. Patients in the study (who were all sixty-five or older) taking SSRIs were more likely to die, suffer a stroke, fall, fracture bones, have a seizure, or experience other adverse effects than those not taking them.

Hyoscyamine (Levsin, Levsinex). Hyoscyamine, an antispasmodic drug, is used to control symptoms associated with disorders of the gastrointestinal tract. It is also used in the treatment of bladder spasms, peptic ulcer disease, diverticulitis, colic, irritable bowel syndrome, cystitis, and pancreatitis. Hyoscyamine may also be used to treat certain heart conditions, to control the symptoms of Parkinson's disease and rhinitis (runny nose), and to reduce excess saliva production.

Hyoscyamine's very strong anticholinergic properties make it inappropriate for older people. Using it to help one problem shuts down so many systems that it always causes serious side effects, including constipation, difficulty urinating, blurred vision, confusion and short-term memory problems, and problems with many other involuntary processes of the body.

Isoxsuprine (Vasodilan). Isoxsuprine is used to relieve the symptoms of central and peripheral vascular diseases such as arteriosclerosis (hardening of the arteries), Buerger's disease (a rare disease of the arteries and veins in the arms and legs), and Raynaud's disease.

In older patients, isoxsuprine's efficacy for its labeled indications is questionable — that is, the drug may not do what the label says it will. No clinical studies have evaluated its safety and effectiveness in patients sixty-five and older, although there is some evidence that it puts elderly patients at higher risk of isoxsuprine-induced hypothermia, which can cause shivering, lethargy, confusion, apathy, delirium, irregular heartbeat, and coma.

Meperidine (Demerol). Meperidine, a narcotic analgesic basically derived from morphine, is used to relieve moderate to severe pain.

Older people are highly sensitive to meperidine and other narcotic drugs. It can build up to toxic levels in an older patient and cause such serious adverse events as arrhythmias, cardiac arrest, slow or troubled breathing, confusion, hallucinations, and orthostatic hypotension. Many safer alternatives are available.

Meprobamate (Miltown, Equanil). Meprobamate, a tranquilizer, is used to treat anxiety disorders or for short-term relief of the symptoms of anxiety.

This is an older drug that's not used as much as it used to be, and for good reason. Its adverse effects include drowsiness, dizziness, and unsteadiness — all of which increase the risk of falls and fractures — as well as cognitive impairment, memory loss, and addiction.

Metaxalone (Skelaxin). Metaxalone, a muscle relaxant, is used to relieve pain and discomfort caused by strains, sprains, and other muscle injuries.

Metaxalone's actual mechanism of action is not known, but it is an inappropriate drug for older people because it can cause anticholinergic side effects, sedation, and weakness. As with cyclobenzaprine (Flexeril), which also appears on the Beers criteria, older patients never should use this drug.

Methocarbamol (Robaxin). Methocarbamol, a muscle relaxant that was first marketed in the United States in 1957, is used to relieve pain and discomfort caused by strains, sprains, and other muscle injuries.

Methocarbamol's actual mechanism of action is not known, but it is inappropriate for older people because it can cause anticholinergic side effects, sedation, and weakness. As with carisoprodol (Soma), which also appears on the Beers criteria, this drug should never be used on older patients.

Methyldopa (Aldomet). Methyldopa, an antihypertensive, is used to treat high blood pressure.

Methyldopa is not used much anymore because it causes so many adverse events, especially in older patients, and especially in those with decreased kidney function or advanced arteriosclerosis.

Mineral oil. Mineral oil is often used to relieve constipation. Although it is often mistakenly referred to as a laxative, it is really just an emollient, or lubricant, that makes the stool slippery so that it can slide more easily through the large intestine. It also retards the colon's absorption of water, softening the stool.

Older people should not use mineral oil. It can decrease the absorption of fat-soluble vitamins and some nutrients. And, once this insoluble oil is consumed, it can be aspirated back up into the esophagus and lungs. Chronic mineral oil aspiration can cause acute and chronic pneumonitis (inflammation of the lungs), localized granulomas (skin lesions), and pulmonary fibrosis, leading, in the worst cases, to death. For this reason, mineral oil has been removed from all laxative products.

Nifedipine (Procardia, Adalat). Nifedipine, a dihydropyridine calcium channel blocker, is used to treat hypertension and to control chest pain from angina. This drug belongs to one of three classes of calcium channel blockers, which differ not only in their basic chemical structure but also in how they relax blood vessels and increase the supply of blood and oxygen to the heart.

Nifedipine comes in both immediate- and controlled-release forms. Although the immediate-release form is frequently prescribed for chronic high blood pressure, it has never been approved by the FDA for that purpose, and since 1996, its labeling has carried a warning that it should not be used to treat high blood pressure. Its use in geriatric patients (those seventy-one years of age and older) has been associated with a nearly fourfold increase in the risk of death from all causes when compared with other antihypertensive drugs, such as nondihydropyridine calcium channel blockers.

Nitrofurantoin (Macrodantin). Nitrofurantoin, an antibacterial drug, is used primarily to treat urinary tract infections. It is an especially bad choice for older patients, however, because it has very high renal-clearance problems.

The kidneys of an average seventy-five-year-old are much less able to clear many types of drugs, including nitrofurantoin, because they're functioning at only about half the efficiency of those of a young adult. That means nitrofurantoin can accumulate steadily in the body, which may cause serious side effects such as anxiety attacks, delusions, and hallucinations; a worsening of existing cardiac problems; a variety of respiratory problems, including interstitial lung disease (scarring of the lung tissue) and pulmonary fibrosis, both of which can be fatal; and hemolytic anemia (a form of anemia caused by the abnormal breakdown of red blood cells), which also can be fatal.

Orphenadrine (Norflex). Orphenadrine, a muscle relaxant, is used to relieve pain and discomfort caused by strains, sprains, and other muscle injuries.

Orphenadrine's actual mechanism of action is not known, but it is an inappropriate drug for older people because it can cause anticholinergic side effects, sedation, and weakness.

Pentazocine (Talwin). Pentazocine, an opiate (narcotic) analgesic, is used to treat pain.

Older adults should not use pentazocine because of its potential for increased central nervous system side effects, including confusion and hallucinations, and drug-induced dependency. Numerous safer drugs are available.

Perphenazine-Amitriptyline (Triavil). This drug combines perphenazine, a conventional antipsychotic used to treat the symptoms of schizophrenia, with amitriptyline, a tricyclic antidepressant that is used to treat symptoms of depression.

Piroxicam (Feldene). Piroxicam, an NSAID, is used to relieve pain, tenderness, swelling, and stiffness caused by osteoarthritis and rheumatoid arthritis.

This NSAID is not prescribed much anymore because of the high incidence of serious and fatal GI bleeds associated with its use. Unfortunately, however, there are still millions of active prescriptions for the drug out there.

Promethazine (Phenergan). Promethazine, a phenothiazine, is most commonly used to control nausea and vomiting. Because of its powerful anticholinergic effects, it's actually classified as a neuroleptic drug.

Older people should not take promethazine for any reason. As an anticholinergic with strong sedative properties, it can cause serious adverse events such as drug-induced parkinsonism (a tremor that's often indistinguishable from Parkinson's disease) and tardive dyskinesia (an irreversible disorder characterized by repetitive, involuntary movements, such as grimacing and tongue thrusting). Along with these problems come the more typical adverse effects of anticholinergics, including constipation, difficulty urinating, blurred vision, confusion and short-term memory problems, and problems with many other involuntary processes of the body.

Propantheline (Pro-Banthine). Propantheline, an anticholinergic drug, is used with other medications to treat ulcers.

This very old drug is not used very much anymore because of its high adverse-event profile. With the introduction of H_2 blockers and proton pump inhibitors, propantheline lost its importance in the treatment of gastrointestinal disorders. Like other highly anticholinergic drugs, it can cause constipation, difficulty urinating, blurred vision, confusion and short-term memory problems, and problems with many other involuntary processes of the body.

Reserpine (Serpalan, Serpasil). Reserpine, a rauwolfia alkaloid, is used to treat high blood pressure. It also is used to treat severe agitation in patients with mental disorders. Although the antihypertensive effects are good, the incidence of depression in patients prescribed the drug makes its use inadvisable.

Ticlopidine (Ticlid). Ticlopidine, a blood-clotting inhibitor, is used to reduce the risk of stroke in people who have had a stroke or have had warning signs of a stroke and who cannot be treated with aspirin. Ticlopidine is also used along with aspirin to prevent blood clots from forming in coronary stents (metal tubes surgically placed in clogged blood vessels to improve blood flow), although this is not an FDA-approved use of the drug.

While ticlopidine is widely prescribed to older patients who are intolerant of — or allergic to — aspirin, it has a high risk of toxicity compared with alternative agents. The drug carries an FDA black-box warning for life-threatening blood disorders. According to one study, more than half the patients on ticlopidine developed adverse gastrointestinal events, including nausea and diarrhea. Older people nearly always experience unwanted effects from taking the drug.

Trimethobenzamide (Tigan). Trimethobenzamide, an antihistamine, is used to treat nausea and vomiting that may occur after surgery. It is also used to control nausea caused by gastroenteritis ("stomach flu").

Although trimethobenzamide has been in

use for a long time, there is little solid evidence that it is effective. Like other highly anticholinergic drugs, it can cause constipation, difficulty urinating, blurred vision, confusion and short-term memory problems, and problems with many other involuntary processes of the body, and it can sometimes cause convulsions.

Tripelennamine (Pyribenzamine). Tripelennamine, a first-generation antihistamine, is a psychoactive drug that is used as an anti-itch medication, or antipruritic. It is also used to treat asthma, hay fever, rhinitis, and urticaria (hives).

Tripelennamine's anticholinergic properties make it inappropriate for use in older patients; adverse effects include constipation, difficulty urinating, blurred vision, confusion and short-term memory problems, and problems with many other involuntary processes of the body.

OFF THE CHARTS: DO YOU REALLY NEED THOSE BLOOD PRESSURE DRUGS?

Hypertension is the most common chronic illness in the United States. Public health officials say that while at least fifty million Americans have blood pressure high enough to warrant medical intervention, only about thirty million of them are being treated for it. And barely more than half of those being treated are able to bring their blood pressure into an acceptable range.

The World Health Organization reports that hypertension is responsible for 49 percent of all ischemic heart disease worldwide and 62 percent of all cerebrovascular disease. Ischemic heart disease — recurring chest pain or discomfort that occurs when the heart muscle doesn't receive enough blood — is the leading cause of death in the United States. Cerebrovascular disease — a group of conditions that affect the flow of blood to the brain — can cause strokes, the third-leading cause of death in the United

States, and a host of other life-threatening health problems.

The prevalence of the disease is not for want of an adequate armamentarium. To most patients (and, shockingly, to many physicians), the array of hypertension drugs on the market is downright bewildering. They include diuretics, adrenergic inhibitors (including alpha-blockers and beta-blockers), direct vasodilators, calcium antagonists, ACE inhibitors, and angiotensin receptor blockers, just to name the major classes of antihypertensives.

If you're older, at some point you're likely to have a doctor tell you that your blood pressure is too high, and, having informed you of that fact, give you a prescription for at least one hypertension drug. Hypertension is the number one diagnosis reported in outpatient medical offices. More than half of all Americans in their sixties are hypertensive, as are three-fourths of those over seventy. Or so the statistics say.

I attach that caveat because I believe the statistics tend to exaggerate the prevalence of hypertension. The reason is simple. The statistics are based largely on the use of antihypertension medications, and in my experience, many patients who are taking these medications don't have high blood pressure at all.

It all has to do with how people get put on these drugs in the first place. Too often it goes like this: they see the doctor for one reason or another, the doctor or a nurse takes their blood pressure, and they leave with a prescription for an antihypertension drug. To base a patient's diagnosis on a single blood pressure reading is, in my judgment, downright irresponsible.

But that's exactly what's happened with more than three of every four patients I see who have been prescribed blood pressure medications, as I can tell from reading their charts. I find this especially troubling because the prescribing doctor generally expects that the patient will stay on the drug, or one like it, and perhaps even additional blood pressure medications, for the rest of his or her life. For all but a few, it's a "forever" prescription that all too often brings with it substantial health risks.

The average person's blood pressure is a little bit like a yo-yo, and a reading taken after an apprehensive or aggravating wait in a doctor's reception room may be seriously misleading. Some people have a fear of doctors — even just sitting in a doctor's office — that artificially elevates their blood pressure. Others get mad because they've been kept waiting for so long, which can have exactly the same result.

Blood pressure is measured in two parts: systolic, when the heart beats while pumping blood; and diastolic, when the heart is at rest between beats. A normal blood pressure level is less than 120/80 mmHg (millimeters of mercury). A high blood pressure level is anything over 140/90 mmHg. In-between readings generally are the basis for a diagnosis of prehypertension.

An average from multiple studies shows that more than 25 percent of people who have elevated blood pressure when someone else takes the reading (generally with an inflatable cuff) actually have a false elevation. The systolic reading averaged 27 mmHg too high, and the diastolic reading, 15 mmHg too high. That's more than enough for a mistaken diagnosis that will put them on medications they don't even need.

Researchers call this type of elevated reading "white-coat hypertension," so named for what the doctors or nurses taking the reading typically wear. One definition of white-coat hypertension is "a conditioned response in some patients that is probably the result of anxiety in the medical setting."

A 2008 statement issued jointly by the

American Heart Association, the American Society of Hypertension, and the Preventive Cardiovascular Nurses Association said: "There is a rapidly growing literature showing that measurements taken by patients at home are often lower than readings taken in the office and closer to the average blood pressure recorded by 24-hour ambulatory monitors, which is the blood pressure that best predicts cardiovascular risk."

For these and other reasons, I insist that patients who see me complete a blood pressure log over two weeks by taking their own blood pressure, along with reading their pulse, first thing in the morning and last thing at night. This should be standard practice before prescribing antihypertension drugs, but, sad to say, it isn't. My educated guess is that fewer than 10 percent of the doctors prescribing these drugs put an at-home blood pressure monitor on their patients or have them take their own readings for a comparable period. They're easy to use, and you take them off after each reading.

This is even harder to understand because there are so many automatic arm and wrist monitors on the market that make getting accurate readings really easy. *Consumer Reports* even rates at-home blood pressure monitors for accuracy and reliability; the models it recently tested ranged in price from $30 to $130. I can't think of a much better investment before you go on a lifelong regimen of antihypertension drugs.

Nor am I alone in recommending this. The American Heart Association, for example, recommends that people with high blood pressure or suspected high blood pressure routinely monitor themselves. And the older you are, the more important it is that you do this, for two main reasons. First, older people have more fluctuations in blood pressure than younger people. A one-shot reading is inherently unreliable. Second, older people are often taking other prescription or over-the-counter medications that raise blood pressure. Examples include acetaminophen, antidepressants, decongestants, and NSAIDs, as well as caffeine and even many herbal supplements.

If you're fifty-five or older, you should own a wristwatch-type blood pressure and pulse monitor. You should take and record your values on a log every night when you go to bed and the first thing in the morning when you get up. This log could save your life. If your values consistently register higher than 140/90, you need to see your doctor for further study as to why. Additionally, if you're taking blood pressure medicine, you can monitor how well it's working for you. Blood pressure values go up and down throughout the day consistent with mood, pain, anxiety, or any external event, and aren't necessarily good indicators of blood pressure problems. But taking and recording your a.m. and p.m. values on a regular basis gives you a pretty firm analysis of what your body is doing.

With all this background out of the way, let's move on to the medications.

THE "FEEL BAD" DRUGS

In my private practice as a pharmacotherapist, I hardly ever meet anyone taking antihypertensive drugs who doesn't complain about the side effects. Sometimes, of course, a person is taking so many different drugs that he or she can't relate the side effects to specific medications. But I certainly can.

Among the most common side effects of blood pressure medications are skin rashes, muscle weakness, dry mouth and eyes, shortness of breath, coughing, lowered energy levels, syncope (fainting), vertigo, and orthostatic hypotension (a sudden drop in blood pressure when a person stands up or stretches). These, especially the last two, are the conditions that people instinctively

166

attribute to their blood pressure medications.

While these may not seem like major health problems, especially compared with other side effects described in this book, they're incredibly significant. They affect what researchers describe as compliance. Studies show that 30 percent to 50 percent of patients stop taking their antihypertensive medications after starting them, and the studies' authors go into great detail exploring factors such as the high cost of the drugs and forgetfulness on the part of the patient. They tend to ignore the one huge, important thing: as a rule, patients really don't like the way blood pressure drugs make them feel.

This, fortunately, is an easily correctable problem that's resolved by matching the blood pressure drug with the patient's lifestyle, organ function, and blood chemistry. The goal is to make the drug do only one job: lowering blood pressure.

Blood pressure medications fall into six basic categories.

Thiazide diuretics. These drugs, sometimes called water pills, work by helping the kidneys to flush excess water and electrolytes from the body, thus lowering blood pressure. They work by inhibiting the reabsorption of sodium in the distal tubule of the kidney. Aside from the undesirable loss of electrolytes, thiazide diuretics typically have fewer side effects than other types of diuretics. Older patients, however, have a problem clearing thiazide diuretics from their bodies because of their reduced renal function. The average person needs to have a creatinine clearance (CrCl) of at least 40 cc/min (cubic centimeters per minute) to ensure that the drug ingested clears the body within twenty-four hours. This complicates the use of thiazide diuretics as antihypertensive agents in older patients. The thiazide is processed in the upper part of the glomeruli (the capillary tufts that filter blood within the kidneys to form urine), and as we age, this part of our filtration system becomes progressively less efficient. Fortunately, another part of each kidney's filtration system, the loop of Henle, takes up the slack, so to speak, but with a few limitations. The limitations can be overcome with loop diuretics, which work a lot better than thiazide diuretics in patients with reduced kidney function.

Alpha-blockers. These drugs, which are also called alpha-adrenergic blocking agents, work by interfering with the transfer of messages to alpha receptors, which are found in blood vessels, in the prostate, and in special blood pressure sensors called baroreceptors. Like other "blocker" medications, they prevent certain hormones — the body's chemical messages — from reaching their targets.

Frequently prescribed alpha-blockers include doxazosin (Cardura), guanfacine (Intuniv), phentolamine (Regitine), tamsulosin (Flomax), and terazosin (Hytrin).

Because alpha-blockers produce a more pronounced dilation, or expansion, of the blood vessels than other drugs, they are fine in a crisis but not good on a routine basis. A lot of falls in older people are attributable to alpha-blockers, especially when the drug is delivered via a sustained-release skin patch, which in and of itself is a huge reason not to prescribe them when alternatives are available. But alpha-blockers can also dysregulate blood sugar control as well as cause dizziness, insomnia, nightmares, and urinary retention, and so their use in older patients needs to be closely monitored.

Beta-blockers. These drugs work by blocking certain nerve and hormonal signals to the heart and to blood vessels throughout the body, causing the heart to beat slower and with less force. With the heart pumping not as much blood through the blood vessels, the pressure against the vessel walls is lowered.

Frequently prescribed beta-blockers include atenolol (Tenormin), carvedilol (Coreg), metoprolol (Lopressor, Toprol XL), nadolol (Corgard), penbutolol (Levatol), and sotalol (Betapace).

When beta-blockers were first introduced, their manufacturers spread around all kinds of misinformation about calcium channel blockers, an older and much less expensive class of drugs used to treat high blood pressure. The drug companies are in business to make money, so I understand why they would do that. But I fault doctors for not taking the time to figure out that what the drug companies were telling them wasn't always the truth.

Beta-blockers are most misprescribed in patients sixty-five or older. In younger patients, they work reasonably well, although in women, common adverse events include various central nervous system problems, including depression, insomnia, and nightmares. These symptoms often aren't identified as side effects of the beta-blocker, with the result that antianxiety, antidepressant, and sedative hypnotic medications are frequently prescribed on top of the offending drug. In older patients, beta-blockers do what they're supposed to do, although perhaps less effectively than other drugs, but they carry a lot of excess baggage in terms of adverse events, including insomnia, Raynaud's disease, muscle pain, joint pain, memory loss, and cognitive changes.

Beta-blockers should not be prescribed to patients with any type of respiratory disease. I've seen older patients with glaucoma have an asthma attack after applying just a single drop of an ophthalmic beta-blocker in an eye. Beta-blockers are also contraindicated in patients with diabetes, as they can cause severe dysregulation of glucose control.

Beta-blockers can also induce depression, and I often see very dramatic instances of this in geriatric patients. And when a patient goes to a psychiatrist because he or she is depressed, do you think that the psychiatrist is going to connect the depression with the beta-blocker? I never see it happen.

Calcium channel blockers. These drugs prevent calcium from entering the muscle cells of the heart and blood vessels, causing the cells to relax and thus lowering blood pressure.

Frequently prescribed calcium channel blockers include amlodipine (Norvasc), diltiazem (Cardizem, Dilacor XR), and nifedipine (Adalat, Procardia).

I generally prefer benzothiazepine calcium channel blockers in older patients. The chief reason is that they are metabolized in the liver by CYP3A4, the most dominant liver enzyme. Because older people, as a rule, have an abundance of CYP3A4, you can predict the outcome of the therapy with much more precision. Although beta-blockers are very popular, if you go to the emergency room with cardiac arrhythmias, the treatment of choice is an IV drip of diltiazem until a normal heart rhythm is maintained. To me, this is added substantiation of the value of the calcium channel blockers.

Angiotensin-converting enzyme (ACE) inhibitors. These drugs work by preventing the body from producing angiotensin II, a hormone that normally causes blood vessels to narrow and, thus, the blood pressure to rise.

Frequently prescribed ACE inhibitors include benazepril (Lotensin), captopril (Capoten), enalapril (Vasotec), lisinopril

(Prinivil, Zestril), quinapril (Accupril), and ramipril (Altace). There's a lot of hype about how these drugs protect the kidneys and heart in diabetic patients. While that may have some merit with younger patients, the reduced renal function of older patients tends to negate all the possible benefits of ACE therapy.

One of the telltale adverse effects of all the ACE inhibitors is a chronic, hacking cough. In my experience, patients are almost never warned about this and are unlikely to associate the cough with their blood pressure medication. Studies suggest that up to a third of all patients taking an ACE inhibitor will develop a chronic cough as a result, and the cough often doesn't go away when they stop taking the drug. This happens more with women than men, and more with African Americans and Asians than others.

ACE inhibitors generally should not be prescribed to African Americans and Asians, in fact, because differences in their renin-angiotensin systems — hormone systems that regulate blood pressure and water balance — lead to dramatically higher incidences of serious adverse events, including angioedema, intestinal angioedema, and the chronic, hacking cough mentioned above.

The intestinal angioedema (a swelling of the muscular bowel wall), a fairly rare condition, is then often misdiagnosed as gastroesophageal reflux disease (GERD) or other GI disorders, with additional drugs prescribed to treat those conditions. In the worst cases, the vocal cords and tongue swell to a point where, if not corrected promptly, they can suffocate the patient.

You might be wondering how a blood pressure drug could cause respiratory problems. These medications affect the process of renal perfusion, which is how the kidneys filter impurities out of the blood. As an older person loses kidney function, the change is reflected in his or her glomerular filtration rate (GFR). The lower your GFR, the more difficult it is for your body to clear drugs from the kidneys and bloodstream, lowering their effectiveness and potentially causing them to accumulate at toxic levels in the body. In this case, the insoluble by-products of the drugs, called kinins, are not filtered out of the blood. They then flow out of the kidneys and lodge themselves in the lungs' bronchial tubes, triggering the chronic dry-coughing spells. Even after the drug is stopped, the cough can linger for months until all the kinins eventually find their way out of the lungs.

. . . .

Angiotensin receptor blockers (ARBs).
These drugs work by blocking the effect of
angiotensin II, a hormone that normally
causes blood vessels to narrow.

Frequently prescribed ARBs include losar-
tan (Cozaar), valsartan (Diovan), losartan-
hydrochlorothiazide (Hyzaar), olmesartan
(Benicar), and telmisartan (Micardis).

ARBs are often prescribed to patients who
are unable to tolerate ACE inhibitors. In
older patients, however, I see few differences
between the two classes of drugs. The positive outcomes sometimes attributed to angiotensin receptor blockers are difficult to
evaluate because two or more other antihypertensives are usually prescribed concurrently. The drug companies have pushed
doctors to prescribe ever-increasing doses
of these drugs in an attempt to generate
positive outcomes. The most worrisome
adverse event associated with ARBs is angioedema, which can rapidly turn into a life-
threatening emergency if the airway becomes blocked.

Like ACE inhibitors, ARBs should generally not be prescribed to African Americans
and Asians because of differences in their

renin-angiotensin systems (see page 173).

The Cochrane Hypertension Review Group, an international network of independent researchers who systematically review various therapies for hypertension, published a comprehensive review of ARBs in 2009; they found the blood pressure–lowering effect of ARBs to be "modest." But the caveat attached to the review is tantamount to a caveat emptor:

Almost all of the trials in this review were funded by companies that make ARBs and serious adverse effects were not reported by the authors of half of these trials. This could mean that the drug companies are withholding unfavorable findings related to their drugs. Due to incomplete reporting of the number of participants who dropped out of the trials due to adverse drug reactions, as well as the short duration of these trials, this review could not provide a good estimate of the harms associated with this class of drugs.

There are lots of questions surrounding the use of blood pressure medications, and often they're not that easy to answer. How can you be sure that you really need to take a drug for hypertension? Which type of drug is right for you? Will your doctor be able to pick the right one? If only your systolic pressure is elevated, should you be taking a drug? Under what circumstances might more than one drug be needed to treat your high blood pressure? Are blood pressure medications really "lifetime drugs"? The list goes on and on.

Many patients wait too long to ask questions. A few years ago, I got a call from an eighty-two-year-old man who kept falling frequently. I suspected that the problem would be related to blood pressure drugs, which have strong sedative effects and often cause dizziness and orthostatic hypotension, which can lead to fainting and falling. Older people are especially prone to this adverse effect because our internal system to regulate blood pressure slows down as we age, and the drug only exacerbates this phenomenon.

When the man came into my office, I took one look at the drugs he was taking — and he was taking them all under the supervision of one doctor — and my jaw dropped. He was on *five* different blood pressure drugs. I could only ask myself, "Why go in there with all these different drugs to do one job?"

177

First off, he was taking a beta-blocker, which generally isn't the best choice for treating hypertension in older adults. That's because nearly half of all people sixty and older don't produce the liver enzyme (CYP2D6) necessary to metabolize the drug properly. As the beta-blocker builds up in a patient's system, all the adverse effects commonly associated with its use are exacerbated, chief among them: insomnia, dizziness, vertigo, and falls. On top of all that, the man was a diabetic, and you're not supposed to take a beta-blocker if you have diabetes because it dysregulates glucose control and normally leads to sudden episodes of hypoglycemia, which can cause blackouts, fainting, and falls.

As with this case, what I see on a daily basis is really pretty scary. I'd say that about 20 percent of my patients who are on blood pressure medications don't need them at all, and that another 50 percent of them are on the wrong type of medication. And about half the time, their blood pressure medications are doing more harm than good.

About 40 percent of the patients I see are on four or more different blood pressure medications, which opens the door to all kinds of life-threatening problems. As a rule of thumb, I want older patients to be taking no more than two blood pressure drugs. The first is generally a benzothiazepine calcium channel blocker such as diltiazem (Cardizem). Then, when we have the diastolic blood pressure in the range we want but the systolic pressure is still too high, adding a low dose of chlorthalidone (Hydone) may be desirable. (If edema is a factor, then a loop diuretic is worth considering.) Although chlorthalidone is a thiazide diuretic, in low doses it lowers the systolic blood pressure without producing a diuretic effect.

Many doctors, however, will put a patient on one drug, then another, then another — adding drugs until they get the patient's blood pressure where they want it (if they ever do). It's therapeutic overkill, because the physician isn't even considering all the harmful interactions that are going on with the unneeded drugs.

Sometimes I really can't figure out what doctors might have been thinking in trying to treat a patient's hypertension, and in some cases, I have to wonder if they even have an idea of the problems that their trial-and-error prescribing methods might be causing.

Keep in mind, too, that it takes many

patients a long time, and a lot of suffering, to question their doctor's competence and search for a consultant pharmacist. Lottie Williams came to see me in 2011 at the urging of her daughter, after she'd apparently begun wondering whether her doctor really knew what he was doing in treating her health issues.

At seventy-three, she was being weighed down by a raft of medical problems, including cardiovascular disease, hypertension, type 2 diabetes, numbness in her extremities, migraine headaches, severe coughing spells, and blackouts that she and her daughter described to me as seizures. She was on eighteen prescription medications, seven of them just for her high blood pressure: an alpha-blocker, two beta-blockers, a long-acting calcium channel blocker, a product that combines an ARB and a thiazide diuretic, a vasodilator, and a loop diuretic.

Right off the bat, I could see that most of her problems were being caused by the blood pressure drugs and the load of the other medications on top of them. Because of her impaired renal clearance, she should not have been put on the alpha-blocker, which placed her at high risk of severe orthostatic hypotension and was undoubtedly a factor in the blackouts. For the same reason, she should not have been prescribed a product containing a thiazide diuretic; these drugs can exacerbate electrolyte problems and hyperglycemia. Because Lottie is African American, she should not have been put on the ARB; African Americans with hypertension respond less favorably to them than whites do. And given her type 2 diabetes, the concomitant use of the two beta-blockers was contraindicated; those drugs were also causing her joint and muscle pains, and the tingling in her fingers was a telltale symptom of beta-blocker-induced Raynaud's disease, which causes smaller arteries that supply blood to your fingers and toes to narrow. Furthermore, because she had a history of migraine headaches, the doctor should not have prescribed a vasodilator for her hypertension; vasodilators can make migraines worse and cause many other very serious adverse events.

I also suspected that the sheer weight of all the drugs was causing Lottie's blackouts and seizure-like episodes. Even though these problems had never been properly evaluated by a specialist, her doctor had somehow seen fit to prescribe the epilepsy drug phenytoin (Dilantin), which in this case deserved an extra level of scrutiny because it can elevate blood sugar. He had also prescribed metformin (Glucophage), an antidiabetes drug, even though its use in patients with impaired renal clearance is contraindicated, as it poses a high risk of lactic acidosis (the buildup of lactic acid in the body), which is usually fatal. Over time, as we weaned Mrs. Williams off the alpha- and beta-blockers (these classes of blood pressure drugs can't just be stopped abruptly without putting the patient at risk of a heart attack, stroke, or, in some cases, kidney failure). I thought there was a good chance that we would find that she didn't actually need the Dilantin.

Studies show that beta-blockers and thiazide diuretics can cause diabetes. An analysis of available clinical trials published in the *Journal of Hypertension* in 2005, for example, concluded that "patients exposed to treatment regimens combining thiazides and beta-blockers are at greater risk of developing diabetes than regimens avoiding this combination of drugs." I could only wonder if that was the case with Lottie Williams.

Mary Bascomb came to see me in early 2009. She was seventy-two and, like Lottie

Williams, struggling with lots of health issues. I could tell that she was scared. She complained of episodes where her body trembled and she had a completely "washed out" feeling. She had pain nearly everywhere, limiting her activities, and said that she felt tired all the time. Her most serious medical conditions were type 2 diabetes and hypertension, as well as anemia, high cholesterol, hypothyroidism, and renal impairment. I could also tell from looking at her labs that she had hyperkalemia, or high blood potassium.

I counted seventeen prescription drugs, along with some vitamin and mineral supplements. Seven were blood pressure medications: a thiazide diuretic, a beta-blocker, a long-acting calcium channel blocker, an ARB, an alpha-adrenergic agonist, a vasodilator, and a direct renin inhibitor, a newer drug that's similar to ACE inhibitors and ARBs.

In my judgment, not one of these blood pressure drugs should have been prescribed to Mrs. Bascomb, let alone all seven. Her renal impairment and uncontrolled diabetes should have ruled out both the thiazide diuretic and the ARB. Her diabetes should have excluded the beta-blocker. Her age should have nixed the renin inhibitor, which probably caused her hyperkalemia. Her known allergy to alpha-blockers should have eliminated the alpha-adrenergic agonist, which from a pharmacological standpoint is akin to an alpha-blocker. Her diabetes also contraindicated the use of an alpha-adrenergic agonist. Her diabetes probably should have also ruled out the vasodilator, which can cause problems with blood sugar control.

That brings us to the short-acting calcium channel blocker — in this instance, immediate-release nifedipine. Mrs. Bascomb's doctor had previously put her on amlodipine, a short-acting calcium channel blocker, but had discontinued it when it became clear that she was allergic to the drug. Why, then, would he put her on another drug in the same family? What's more, the use of immediate-release nifedipine in patients of Mrs. Bascomb's age, when compared with short-acting calcium channel blockers, has been associated with a nearly fourfold increase in the risk of death from all causes. All considered, I thought, a puzzling choice for treating her hypertension.

The track record with the other drugs wasn't any better. In an effort to correct her severe anemia, she was taking injections of epoetin alfa (Procrit), a medication used to stimulate the bone marrow to make red blood cells. At 8.9, her hemoglobin (Hgb) was too low to use this drug. (Iron stores have to be increased to bring the Hgb up to at least 10 before the Procrit will work.) Her diabetes would require insulin, since the oral medications were not helping her at all.

All told, I recommended that fourteen of the seventeen prescription drugs Mrs. Bascomb was taking be stopped at once, including the statin drugs that had been prescribed for her high cholesterol, with the remaining three — all of them blood pressure medications — tapered down until they could be discontinued safely. To return her to good health, she went on Venofer, an IV iron injection, to improve her Hgb; diltiazem CD, a calcium channel blocker, and the diuretic chlorthalidone, for her high blood pressure; Lantus, a form of manmade insulin, for her diabetes; and a combination of vitamin B_{12} injections, folic acid, and vitamin B_6 for her high cholesterol.

In pretty short order, freed from nearly all the problems her old medications had been causing, Mrs. Bascomb seemed like a new person. The next time I saw her, I could barely believe the change in her mood, energy level, and outlook. Appropriate drug therapy made all the difference.

THE DRUG-FREE APPROACH

The vast majority of my older patients who have been told that they have high blood pressure — maybe as many as nine out of ten — are going to be on an alpha-blocker, a beta-blocker, and an ACE inhibitor and/or an ARB. This suggests that very, very few doctors are prescribing hypertension drugs appropriately — at least, not when it comes to their older patients.

As I see it, alpha-blockers or beta-blockers should be used only as a last resort. As noted above, both classes of drugs dysregulate glucose control, making them inappropriate for diabetics, other people with blood sugar problems, and patients with respiratory diseases. But many doctors aren't aware of these limitations and prescribe them anyway.

ACE inhibitors and ARBs work in pretty much the same way, although ARBs are a little more sophisticated. Both types of drugs elevate potassium levels in the blood, which can cause hyperkalemia. Symptoms of hyperkalemia generally include malaise, palpitations, and muscle weakness, and, in some cases, mild hyperventilation. Hyperkalemia itself is a medical emergency, as it can lead to abnormal heart rhythms or sudden death. ACE inhibitors and ARBs also cause fatigue and dizziness, which can bring about falls, and also may trigger serious respiratory distress.

With the blood pressure medications, I often see doctors giving more and more and more of a drug, or multiple drugs in the same class, because the desired result hasn't been achieved. The problem doesn't have anything to do with the medications, though, but with the patient's renal system, which can't clear the drugs from the body, or with a lack of the liver chemistry needed to metabolize the drug properly.

In older patients, the doctor then often pushes the issue by increasing the dose or combining it with other drugs. That's the wrong thing to do.

A recent study found that older patients taking both an ACE inhibitor and an ARB, in fact, were 2.4 times as likely to experience kidney failure or to die within six months of starting treatment as those taking just one of the drugs. They were also twice as likely to develop hyperkalemia.

It's shocking to me that we have no randomized controlled trials — clinical studies that are the gold standard of medical research — that look at the adverse effects of using drugs to get blood pressure lower than 140/90, even though they've been prescribed by the millions for decades. What was perhaps the most comprehensive study demonstrated no benefit at all for lower blood pressure targets and failed to report adverse-event data — a shortcoming explained, in all likelihood, by the fact that it was funded by the pharmaceutical industry. And even though the trial enrolled participants up to the age of eighty, no data by age group were presented, making it all but impossible to sort out the potential benefits and risks of the drug therapy in older people. Because antihypertensive drugs can be so dangerous, I urge patients to try controlling their blood pressure through some basic lifestyle changes.

If you are overweight or obese, for example, you can lower your blood pressure (by up to 15 percent, some studies show) simply by losing weight. Perhaps I shouldn't say "simply," as I know how difficult it is for many people to lose weight and not regain it. But the side effects of many of the blood pressure drugs — including depression and impotence and sexual dysfunction — can certainly be a strong motivating factor.

Going hand in hand with weight loss are reducing your intake of salt and fat and increasing the amount of fiber in your diet. Would you rather take a blood pressure drug for the rest of your life or reduce your sodium intake to no more than 1,600 milligrams a day? A study published in the *New England Journal of Medicine* in 2001 found that the two approaches will have about the same effects on blood pressure. Decreasing the amount of animal fat in your diet will also help to lower your blood pressure, as will increasing the fiber in your diet. A major study of nondrug therapies for hypertension found that diets high in fiber can lower blood pressure.

Then come alcohol and tobacco. Both cause irreversible vascular damage, and the older you get, the more damage there will be. Cutting your alcohol intake to one drink a day or less can reduce your blood pressure. And if you smoke cigarettes or use tobacco in any other way, my advice would be to stop now, no matter how many times you've tried before and how difficult it may seem.

Finally, there's exercise. Walking your dog fifteen or twenty minutes a day at a comfortable pace will have a beneficial effect on your blood pressure, as will any kind of walking. A little exercise will also do wonders for joint aches and pain, muscle pains, respiration, and multitudes of other chronic problems seen in the older patient.

And, best of all, these approaches offer something that the drugs can't: a cure for hypertension.

PHANTOM KILLERS: NSAIDs (NONSTEROIDAL ANTI-INFLAMMATORY DRUGS)

Nonsteroidal anti-inflammatory drugs — NSAIDs for short — are one of the most dangerous classes of drugs for older people. NSAIDs are typically used to treat arthritis, joint pain, headaches, and other kinds of pain. They're available in prescription and over-the-counter forms, and there are so many different NSAIDS, marketed in so many different ways, that patients often don't even know that they're using them. Although NSAIDs share broadly similar properties, there are significant differences in how they are taken, how well they are tolerated, and how long they last in the body.

The main problems with NSAIDs are that they increase gastrointestinal irritation (which can lead to erosion of the protective lining of the stomach), assist in the formation of GI bleeds, and decrease the cohesive properties of platelets that are needed to form blood clots. What's more, the regular use of NSAIDs can cause cardiovascular disease.

As early as a decade ago, a research team at Stanford University reported in the *New England Journal of Medicine* that approximately 107,000 people are hospitalized every year for NSAID-related gastrointestinal complications and that at least 16,500 NSAID-related deaths occur each year among arthritis patients.

These statistics, while shockingly high, do not even take into account the use of over-the-counter NSAIDs — among them ibuprofen (Advil, Motrin) and naproxen (Aleve) — that have the same active ingredients as their prescription counterparts.

If you have some form of arthritis, you're already in a high-risk group. More than 14 million Americans with arthritic conditions use NSAIDs on a regular basis. Studies show that up to 60 percent of them will experience adverse gastrointestinal effects related to the NSAIDs they take, and that more than 10 percent will stop taking the medications their doctors have prescribed or recommended because of troublesome GI symptoms.

Apply those percentages to the numbers of Americans taking NSAIDs, and you've got at least 8.4 million people who experience adverse GI effects from the drugs and at least 1.4 million who just stop taking them because of those effects.

The simple fact is that all NSAIDs can cause gastrointestinal toxicity that can lead to GI bleeding and even death. The risk goes up with age, with dose, and with duration of treatment. So if you're an older person who's been taking NSAIDs for a while — or if you've been taking pain medications without knowing whether or not they're NSAIDs — you'd do well to take stock of your NSAID use right away.

I think of NSAIDs as "phantom killers" because people who take them can seriously damage their intestinal lining without even being aware of it, and there can be significant GI bleeding without any symptoms being present. People taking NSAIDs will frequently have blood in their stool but not be able to see it.

Signs of an active GI bleed can include nosebleeds; bleeding gums; cola- or tea-colored urine (hematuria); bloody or black, tarry stools; spitting up blood; or coughing up or vomiting blood or material that looks like coffee grounds (hemoptysis). NSAID-induced bleeding in the stomach or intestines can occur at any time and without any warning. It's one of the scariest things I see on a day-to-day basis.

Many of the patients I see have trouble understanding how what seems like such a simple pain reliever could cause such serious gastrointestinal bleeding. It all begins with the fact that NSAIDs reduce the secretion of gastric mucus, thus inhibiting the formation of the stomach's protective lining. (Studies suggest that different NSAIDs reduce gastric mucus to varying degrees, which may help explain why these drugs can have slightly different GI-toxicity profiles.)

Add to that a simple fact of aging: in an older person, everything is slowing down. Because your stomach isn't producing as much acid as it once did, your body doesn't need to secrete as much gastric mucus to protect it. In short, your stomach's protective mucous membrane lining is thinning as you age, leaving it more vulnerable to the effects of NSAIDs.

As I see it, if you take too many NSAIDs, or take NSAIDs for too long, you're putting yourself on a nearly certain path to stomach problems. One study, for example, showed that 71 percent of subjects who used NSAIDs had an injury in their small intestine, compared with 5 percent of subjects who didn't use NSAIDs.

The GI tract isn't the only system of the body that can be damaged by NSAIDs. People with reduced liver and kidney function also face an elevated risk of renal damage if they take NSAIDs, because their kidneys are not able to excrete the drug adequately.

Here the chemistry has to do with the enzymes in the liver that metabolize the NSAID. Most nonsteroidals are highly protein bound, meaning that as they are absorbed in the body, they attach onto proteins such as albumin, which is in blood. Older people are more prone to complications from NSAIDs because their renal function is impaired.

NSAIDs can also damage your heart. The latest studies show that *all* NSAIDs can increase your blood pressure and put you at increased risk of heart attack, heart failure, stroke, arterial aneurysm, and other adverse cardiovascular events. A study published in the *Archives of Internal Medicine* in 2007, for example, showed that men who took NSAIDs six or seven times a week were 38 percent more likely to develop high blood pressure than those who took no NSAIDs.

This comes about because NSAIDs lead

to prostaglandin inhibition. Prostaglandins are derivatives of fatty acids that influence a variety of processes in the body, including muscle growth. Because prostaglandins are in the heart muscles, just like they are elsewhere, if your body isn't clearing the NSAID properly, the drug is in effect increasing your blood pressure. I don't think that most doctors who prescribe NSAIDs know that.

Nor do they generally know that NSAIDs, in addition to increasing a patient's blood pressure, can actually counteract the effects of the hypertension drugs that have been prescribed. A study published in the journal *Hypertension* in 2007, for example, found calcium channel blockers to be the only exception.

The average patient doesn't know this either, which can lead to all kinds of problems on the blood pressure front. But that's still just the tip of the iceberg.

NSAIDs, as I see it, pose what really amounts to a major public health problem in the United States. In addition to the statistics presented above, consider for a moment that NSAIDs account for 43 percent of all drug-related visits to hospital emergency rooms.

Many, if not most, of these medical emergencies are avoidable. A 2001 study estimated, by reviewing physician and prescription records, that 42 percent of emergency room visits were precipitated by NSAIDs that were prescribed unnecessarily.

That's not counting the millions of Americans who buy NSAIDs over the counter. There are plenty to choose from; in fact, you'll often find an entire aisle of them in the drugstore.

Because people use NSAIDs for so many different purposes — to treat pain and fever from a cold or other illness, for example; or for headaches, muscle pain, menstrual cramps, and all kinds of everyday aches and pains — they can often be taking several different NSAIDs without even realizing it.

They can also achieve or exceed the effect of a prescription-strength NSAID simply by taking more than a single dose of it in over-the-counter form. You need a doctor's prescription to get 400-milligram tablets of ibuprofen, but you can go to your local drugstore or supermarket and buy as many 200-milligram tablets as you want without a prescription. To my way of thinking, that's absurd.

Take an older person with knee pain, for example. He can simply reach into the medicine cabinet and double up the dose on his own. This obviously can be dangerous, especially if it becomes a habit.

With over-the-counter NSAIDs, as with aspirin, the problem arises when people think that if one will do the job, two will do a better job, and three will do an even better job.

Because NSAIDs are so dangerous, if it were up to me, they wouldn't even be available over the counter — or, at least, they'd be required to carry much bigger warnings than they do now.

I see an awful lot of NSAID-related problems when people come to see me for a drug therapy consultation or when I'm reviewing a patient's chart for the first time in a nursing home.

It's important to remember that, along with the inflammation from arthritis, older people also suffer from joint immobility. When a joint doesn't move freely, you hurt. A joint that hasn't been moved sufficiently, in fact, will begin to stiffen within twenty-four hours and will eventually become inflexible.

This is the problem, generally, in people who do not, or cannot, exercise regularly. This includes people with sedentary lifestyles, people in nursing homes and other institutional settings, and people with depression or physical disabilities that limit their mobility. When they experience immobility in their joints, and the pain that goes along with it, the use of an NSAID is overkill. It places the patient at a high risk for serious problems, when a general analgesic such as acetaminophen would have done the job just fine. But I see case after case where doctors don't understand the difference between immobility and inflammation and prescribe NSAIDs anyway.

I also see lots of capillary fragility. That's when the tiny blood vessels right under the skin rupture, leaving tiny red or purple spots or large bruises. Capillary fragility is almost always drug related, and NSAIDs are the most frequent cause.

When I see patients who are using one or more NSAIDs, either in prescription or over-the-counter form, the first thing I look at are the risk factors that can point to additional problems. These are the ones I typically zero in on:

Age. Older people tend to take pain medications more often, or in larger doses, and often in combination with other powerful drugs, than younger people. And because older people are more likely to have reduced liver and kidney function, they should take NSAIDs in lower doses than younger people, if they take them at all. And, really, they *shouldn't* take them at all, as so many non-NSAID analgesics are available that work just as well.

Stomach or intestinal problems. Previous ulcers or other GI problems, such as diverticulitis and Crohn's disease, are another major risk factor and should often rule out the use of NSAIDs.

Alcohol use. Alcohol, on its own, can irritate the gastrointestinal tract. The concurrent use of NSAIDs and alcohol significantly increases the risk of damage to the intestinal lining, including ulcers and GI bleeding, according to a study published in the *American Journal of Gastroenterology* in 1999.

Way back in 1993, the Food and Drug Administration's Nonprescription Drug Advisory Committee recommended that all over-the-counter pain relievers contain an alcohol warning, but some manufacturers — nearly twenty years later — still have not complied. Chronic heavy alcohol users may be at increased risk of liver toxicity from NSAID use.

Corticosteroid use. Corticosteroids are prescribed for arthritis, colitis, and a host of other conditions. In my experience, in fact, doctors will prescribe steroids for just about anything. Studies show that people taking corticosteroids such as prednisone (Deltasone) in doses over 10 milligrams in combination with NSAIDs increase their risk of GI bleeding sevenfold. The danger stems from the fact that NSAIDs are chemical copycats of steroids.

Anticoagulant use. Studies have found that people who use NSAIDs at the same time they are taking oral prescription anticoagulants — like warfarin (Coumadin), for example — have a twelvefold risk of GI bleeding. Why? As the NSAID opens up new avenues for bleeding in the GI tract, the warfarin keeps the blood from clotting. This typically happens when patients who have been prescribed Coumadin by a cardiologist start taking NSAIDs they buy over the counter, but I have seen doctors prescribe them together too.

At first, the COX-2 inhibitors — rofecoxib (Vioxx), celecoxib (Celebrex), and valdecoxib (Bextra) — were advertised as being safe when used with warfarin, but that turned out to be wrong. In fact, in time, all the adverse events seen with NSAIDs were also seen with the COX-2 inhibitors, and the COX-2 inhibitors proved to cause even more cardiovascular problems than the old NSAIDs.

The FDA has recently approved newer anticoagulant medications that also should not be taken with NSAIDs. These include dabigatran (Pradaxa) and rivaroxaban (Xarelto).

I was working in my office one day in 2006 when James Tisdale called and asked to speak with me. The telephone had been ringing quite a bit that morning, as the *Griffin Daily News* had published a front-page story about me and my practice the previous day. As I took the call, I could tell that the man was crying. He told me that he was scared that he was dying and that nobody seemed to know what was wrong with him. He said he'd been sent home that day from physical therapy because he couldn't stand up to do any of the exercises. We made an appointment for the next afternoon. I asked him to stop by my office right away, though, so that he could pick up a copy of the physician referral form that I use, have his doctor fill it out, and bring the completed form with him to the appointment.

When Mr. Tisdale came in the following day, he explained with some embarrassment that he didn't have the referral form. His doctor had refused to fill it out, he said, telling him that she didn't need any help practicing medicine. Then he'd gone to his neurologist, who also refused, saying, "What could a pharmacist possibly tell me about patient care?"

Mr. Tisdale, who owned his own dump-truck company, was seventy-one. Sometime earlier, his primary physician had diagnosed him with arthritis and started him on NSAIDs. When his condition grew worse rather than better, she sent him to the neurologist, who in turn had diagnosed him as having peripheral neuropathy (a nerve condition that often causes numbness, tingling, and pain in the hands and feet) and arthralgia (joint pain) and prescribed three different anticonvulsant drugs for him to take concurrently. His condition worsened even further.

On questioning Mr. Tisdale, I learned that he had also been on several statin drugs over the past year, including, most recently, rosuvastatin (Crestor). He had been experiencing such severe muscle and joint pain, especially in his legs and hips, that he was taking large amounts of acetaminophen throughout the day, in the forms of Arthritis Strength Tylenol and Tylenol PM at night. As I added up his total daily intake, I could see that it easily topped 4,000 milligrams — way above the upper safety parameter of 3,000 milligrams daily. Additionally, on the advice of the nurse in his doctor's office, he'd started taking 400 milligrams of naproxen sodium twice a day for pain. All this in a patient whose creatinine clearance of 47 cc/min should have ruled out NSAIDs altogether.

Mr. Tisdale immediately went to see another doctor with whom I enjoy a good working relationship. We discontinued the NSAIDs immediately and in the weeks ahead adjusted his other medications.

When he came in with his wife two months later for a follow-up visit, he had no problems walking, sitting, or standing. He did scare me, though, when all of a sudden he dropped to the floor without explanation or warning. But just as quickly, he popped back up, with a big grin on his face; he'd just wanted to demonstrate that he was back to his old limber self. I asked him if he was driving his truck again, and he replied that he was back driving full-time. I asked him if he had any leg pain while driving. "Only toward the end of the day," he replied. Then his wife interrupted: "But he's driving ten and eleven hours a day!"

Mr. Tisdale, incidentally, was also happy for another reason: we'd reduced his prescription drug bills by about $800 a month.

All NSAIDs — from Vioxx, which was removed from the market in 2004, to its myriad chemical cousins, which are still on the market — eventually cause cardiovascular disease. Despite the manufacturer-sponsored studies that show NSAIDs to be safe, they clearly are not.

Billed as "super-aspirins" when they were approved by the FDA in 1999, Vioxx and Celebrex were both heavily advertised and promoted by their manufacturers (Merck spent $161 million on direct-to-consumer ads for Vioxx in 2000 alone). The marketing campaign was so successful, in fact, that by 2001, nearly two-thirds of all prescriptions for NSAIDs written during outpatient visits to doctors and hospitals were for Vioxx or Celebrex. In two years, both drugs had achieved "blockbuster" status by generating more than $1 billion in revenue annually.

Merck pulled Vioxx from the market on September 30, 2004, after a company-sponsored clinical trial found more heart attacks and strokes in patients who took the drug than in those taking a placebo (a look-alike that contains no medication). At the time that Vioxx was withdrawn, according to the FDA, two million Americans were taking it.

Pfizer, the manufacturer of Celebrex, went to great lengths to assure consumers that its product didn't carry the same risks. Just a few months later, however, the company announced that Celebrex was also linked to heart attack and stroke. In December 2004 it stopped advertising Celebrex, but sixteen months later, in 2006, it resumed running television and print ads for the drug. All advertising for Celebrex now contains a black-box warning stating that the drug may increase the risk of heart attacks, strokes, blood clots, stomach bleeding, and ulcers. Similarly, G. D. Searle and Company, which manufactured and marketed a similar NSAID, valdecoxib, under the brand name Bextra, removed it from the market in 2005 after the FDA warned that its use was associated with an increased risk of heart attack and stroke.

More than a decade ago, a team of doctors from Stanford University, writing in the *New England Journal of Medicine,* noted that the toxic effects of NSAIDs remained "mainly a 'silent epidemic,' with many physicians and most patients unaware of the magnitude of the problem." Sadly, the problem has gotten worse, not better.

Today some sixty million Americans use NSAIDs on a regular basis. Most of them, researchers have found, develop erosions in their stomachs after each dose. On average, 15 percent to 25 percent of them, if examined with an endoscope (an instrument with a flexible tube that's used to examine the digestive tract), will be found to have developed a discrete — though usually small — ulcer from their regular use of NSAIDs. That's in the neighborhood of fifteen million NSAID-induced ulcers.

It's important to remember, too, that the adverse gastrointestinal effects aren't rare or even unusual. Up to half of all people who take NSAIDs, in fact, have some type of GI distress afterward. And serious gastrointestinal problems often come without warning. It's estimated, in fact, that 80 percent of the people who are affected with serious NSAID-induced GI complications have had no prior symptoms or warning signals.

And even when patients suffer those serious complications, their doctors often don't recognize them.

In 2010 Joe Brown, a seventy-eight-year-old retired air force pilot in San Antonio, Texas, found his way to me. He was in serious trouble. Among his problems: atrial fibrillation (an abnormal heart rhythm) that wasn't being properly treated, diabetes that was interacting with every medication and condition he had, and a rare blood disease that, in the opinion of the hematologist (a specialist in blood diseases) who'd rendered the diagnosis, put him in line for a bone marrow transplant.

As I looked over the twenty prescription drugs that Mr. Brown was taking, I was alarmed to see that he'd been put on high doses of two NSAIDs — indomethacin (Indocin) and meloxicam (Mobic) — that are contraindicated in older patients. No one, apparently, recognized that the NSAIDs were causing his horrible gastrointestinal bleeding. Making matters far worse, his cardiologist had him on warfarin, an anticoagulant that is known to increase the severity of NSAID-induced GI bleeding. The response of the doctors to the GI bleeding was to keep giving Mr. Brown blood transfusions. As a result, his hemoglobin count was so low that he was barely able to stand and had lost the strength, really, to do just about anything.

The specialists who were helping to treat Mr. Brown weren't pleased that he had seen me, to put it mildly. The cardiologist said that he wasn't about to listen to "an Internet pharmacist who doesn't know what he's talking about," as Mr. Brown later related the remark to me. The hematologist simply told Mr. Brown that he knew what he was doing.

Fortunately, Mr. Brown's primary care physician was amenable to discontinuing the two NSAIDs and some other medications (including two statin drugs that may have been causing much of the muscle and joint pain that in turn led to the prescription of the NSAIDs), and to slowly tapering him off pantoprazole (Protonix), a proton pump inhibitor that had been prescribed to help deal with the GI toxicity of the NSAIDs. In time, Mr. Brown was feeling much better, and his hemoglobin was the highest it had been in years. He didn't need any more blood transfusions, and so far he's done fine without the services of the hematologist.

Mr. Brown and his wife are traveling all over the country again, just as they had done before the NSAIDs all but killed him.

He's taking just a few prescription drugs now, including tramadol (Ultram), an analgesic, and an occasional acetaminophen instead of the NSAIDs. With the statins gone, most of his muscle and joint pains have disappeared.

Do you believe that a seemingly innocuous television commercial for an over-the-counter medication can end up killing people? I do, and I'll explain why in giving you this example.

As we were finishing this book, I turned on the television one evening to see Regis Philbin, the famous TV personality, in a new commercial for Advil. It showed Regis and his wife, Joy, playing tennis. "We love to play tennis, and with it come some aches and pains," he said. "And one way to relieve them all is to go right to the Advil. Tennis is our game, and Advil has become part of our game." The commercial closes with an announcer saying, "Take action. Take Advil."

A few days later, I saw another television commercial for Advil with Regis and Joy, this one just a bit longer, with her saying, "I have become increasingly amazed at Regis's endurance. It's scary sometimes what he accomplishes in a day." He then adds, "Well, I'd rather not have time for pain, but unfortunately it does come your way every now and then. And that's when I take my Advil." The commercial closes with the announcer voicing the same tagline.

At first I didn't notice a little line of type in the commercial that said, "Ask a doctor if you are age sixty or over," and I'm pretty sure that's just the way that Pfizer, the manufacturer of Advil, intended. Older people, after all, should not be taking Advil — or any other NSAID.

That goes for Regis Philbin, who was eighty at the time the commercial went on the air, and for his wife, who was seventy. But you can be sure that in selecting this famous couple to launch its "True Advil Stories" campaign, Pfizer was aiming squarely for an older target market that it knows, with certainty, is most susceptible to being harmed by its product.

To me, this is a public deception that should be stopped. I really do wonder how many older people who watch this commercial and do what Regis recommends will eventually end up in the hospital — or six feet under.

Proton Pump Inhibitors: The Miracle Drugs That Aren't

If you've been told that you have gastroe-sophageal reflux disease, or you've decided on your own that you have GERD, as it's often called, join the club. It's a large club that, over the past decade, has experienced a huge surge in membership. Much of the club's rapid growth has been driven by the manufacturers of drugs that are used to treat GERD: they've brought untold millions of Americans into the fold with magazine ads and television commercials that promise quick relief for the indigestion and other gastrointestinal symptoms that nearly all of us experience at one time or another. Maybe you're one of them.

Before the modern generation of acid-suppressing drugs came along, most stomach-acid problems were typically treated with Maalox, Phillips' Milk of Magnesia, and other magnesium-hydroxide preparations. Prescription drugs were used too, including atropine, hyoscyamine (Levsin), scopolamine (Scopace), and other belladonna alkaloids, all of them highly anticholinergic and highly inappropriate for older patients; phenobarbital (Solfoton), a sedative; and muscarinic anticholinergics such as dicyclomine (Bentyl), all of which worked by relaxing the smooth circular muscles that make up the gastrointestinal tract and slowing the production of gastric secretions. As anticholinergics, they caused all kinds of problems in older patients, including extreme constipation, blurred vision, the exacerbation of glaucoma-related problems, urinary retention, confusion, and hallucinations.

While scientists were aware that the secretion of stomach acid was triggered by histamine, they also knew that traditional antihistamines didn't work for this purpose. Researchers at Smith Kline & French (now GlaxoSmithKline), correctly postulating that another kind of histamine receptor controlled the secretion of stomach acid, named this second receptor H_2 and went on to develop a drug to block it.

This drug was cimetidine, the first histamine H_2 receptor antagonist (or histamine-2 blocker, or H_2 blocker). It debuted in 1976 under the brand name Tagamet and soon became the first-ever "blockbuster drug." Cimetidine is so powerful, however, that over time it will essentially shut down the patient's liver, with the result that any other drug he or she takes won't work so well or won't work at all.

To address that problem, researchers kept working to modify the drug, and in time other H_2 blockers were developed from cimetidine, including famotidine (Pepcid), nizatidine (Axid), and ranitidine (Zantac). Today all of these prescription medications are also available over the counter.

The development of the H_2 blockers was really a big step forward in the treatment of stomach disorders, especially gastric disorders, because for the first time, you could actually slow down the production of acid.

Three years after Tagamet was introduced, scientists discovered omeprazole, the first of a new class of more powerful drugs to control the secretion of acid in the stomach. It was called a proton pump inhibitor (PPI), as it inhibited the gastric acid pump. Omeprazole was first marketed in 1988 under the brand name Prilosec, and it too led to the development of other PPIs, including lansoprazole (Prevacid), pantoprazole (Protonix), and rabeprazole (Aciphex). In 2001 came esomeprazole (Nexium), the fifth PPI to reach the market.

PPIs are approved for the treatment of GERD as well as gastric ulcers, erosive esophagitis, and GI bleeds associated with the use of nonsteroidal anti-inflammatory drugs (NSAIDs).

Today proton pump inhibitors are thought to be the second-best-selling class of medications in the world. Unfortunately, they are also one of the most dangerous and misunderstood.

Let's start with a few basics about proton pump inhibitors. If you're taking a PPI for acid reflux, you probably don't need to be. If you were started on a PPI in the hospital, chances are that you never needed the drug in the first place. If you've been taking a PPI for a long time to treat acid reflux or GERD, either you or your doctor is going off label and using it for a purpose that's not been approved by the Food and Drug Administration (FDA). If you're older, you're taking a drug that's never been studied in your age group. And if you or your doctor decides at some point to stop the PPI therapy, you're likely to find the process of getting off the drug to be very difficult if not impossible.

Now for the worst of the news: long-term

use of proton pump inhibitors has been associated with a variety of intestinal infections (including the bacterium *C. difficile,* which can be fatal), pneumonia, certain types of stomach cancers, bone fractures, vitamin B_{12} deficiencies, other vitamin and mineral deficiencies, and a host of other serious adverse effects.

To understand how PPIs work and how they can cause so many different problems, a look at some of the basic forces at play may be helpful.

To begin with, gastroesophageal reflux (GER) is just the four-dollar word for acid reflux or acid regurgitation, which is what happens when digestive juices — stomach acids — flow up into the esophagus. Normally this is prevented by the lower esophageal sphincter (LES), a muscular valve between the esophagus and the stomach. Acid reflux can occur when this valve malfunctions, typically by opening when it's not supposed to or by not sealing properly when it closes. This is especially common among older people, whose lower esophageal sphincter is more likely to become too relaxed or weak.

One of the telltale signs of acid reflux is that you can taste food or stomach fluid in the back of your throat. Another is the burning sensation in your chest or throat that's caused by refluxed stomach acid coming into contact with the lining of your esophagus — the condition commonly called heartburn or acid indigestion.

Occasional gastroesophageal reflux is common and doesn't necessarily mean that you have GERD, which is *GER* with a *D* added for disease. The line between GER and GERD can be an extremely fuzzy one, with one popular definition for GERD being "troublesome symptoms and/or complications" brought on by acid reflux and another being the occurrence of heartburn or acid reflux at least twice a week. With two out of five people reporting heartburn or acid reflux at least once a month, it's easy to see why prescription pads get pulled out so often — and why so many people skip that step and self-medicate with over-the-counter products.

Studies show that at least half, and possibly more than two-thirds, of all people taking PPIs don't even have a condition that the drugs are designed to treat. That's an especially alarming statistic when you consider that more than 119 million prescriptions for proton pump inhibitors were written in the United States in 2009, accounting for $13.6 billion in sales. If you go to your doctor with gastrointestinal complaints, studies show, you're more likely to be diagnosed with GERD than any other condition.

While PPIs have been tested and approved only for short-term treatment of GERD, studies also show that many people take these drugs for much longer periods of time. Many of the patients who come to see me, in fact, have been on prescription-strength PPIs for years, and most of them see it not as a short-term therapeutic intervention but as a "lifetime" drug.

The biggest problem with PPIs is what happens when you try to stop taking them. Studies show that people who take PPIs for a month or more and then stop make even more stomach acid than before they started taking the drug. This phenomenon is known as rebound acid hypersecretion, and it's caused as the body jacks up the production of gastric acid in an effort to return the stomach to its natural, pre-PPI pH level. As the acid reflux symptoms return with a vengeance, most patients ("nearly all," according to one review of the available studies) begin taking the PPI again and thus start down the road to long-term drug dependence. This is a particularly painful and dangerous outcome for the large number of people who shouldn't even have been prescribed PPIs in the first place.

Worse yet, if you didn't have GERD when you started out on a PPI, you may well have it before you're finished. A team of researchers in the Netherlands, as part of a study published in the journal *Gastroenterology* in 2009, put people with no symptoms of GERD on PPI therapy for six weeks. At the end of the six-week study, every participant had symptoms of GERD.

In a letter to the FDA in 2011 in support of black-box warnings on PPIs, journalist Robert Kuttner, a longtime columnist for *BusinessWeek* and coeditor of the *American Prospect,* recounted his experiences taking the drugs as a "68-year-old male in generally good health" and "longtime sufferer of severe gastroesophageal reflux disease."

Soon after a 1993 visit to the emergency room landed him a referral to a gastroenterologist, Kuttner was started on what became a daily maintenance dose (20 milligrams) of omeprazole (Prilosec). But over time, Kuttner wrote, the acid-reflux attacks — some of them just like the one that sent him to the ER — seemed to be triggered more easily. Here, in Kuttner's own words, is the next part of the story:

Whenever these bouts occurred — maybe six or eight times a year — my doctor recommended tripling the dose of Prilosec for a week or two to calm things down, then gradually tapering back to my normal dose. When I tried to taper the dose more abruptly, I experienced repeat attacks, more frequent and sometimes stronger than before. Over time, I became progressively reliant on higher doses for longer periods of time. At no point did I attempt to stop the PPI "cold turkey" for fear of even stronger reactions.

The doctor and I concluded that all this was a somewhat inexplicable, worsening propensity to GERD, possibly due to less efficient containment of stomach acid. We did not address the possibility of chronic rebound effects from the medication.

In time, Kuttner was, at the suggestion of his gastroenterologist, taking as much as 80 milligrams of Prilosec a day. In 2010, after reading some studies that Sidney M. Wolfe, MD, the director of Public Citizen's Health Research Group, had shared with him, Kuttner concluded that his progressively worsening condition might have been caused by the Prilosec. His internist referred him to another gastroenterologist, who agreed to work with him to end his dependence on the drug. Kuttner's letter to the FDA concluded with these observations:

My experience certainly seems to confirm the pattern of PPI medication causing — or, in my case, seriously aggravating — the condition that it supposedly treats. In my case, the PPI seemed to have primed my system to produce increasing amounts of acid so that over time I was more prone to more attacks triggered by ever more minor departures from a very low-fat diet. The ever-increasing amounts of PPI helped only temporarily and required dependence on even higher doses, and so on, over several cycles.

Only getting off the PPI reversed what seemed to be a chronic and progressive condition [emphasis in original].

Over the years, I've seen what Robert Kuttner lived through more times than I'd like to remember. In older people, a PPI is nearly always the wrong drug for acid reflux. When it comes to acid reflux, my philosophy is to fight it when you have it, not to fight it all the time. Because when you put a patient on a proton pump inhibitor indefinitely, you never allow the stomach to reset its computer, so to speak. Besides, a PPI is really a short-term drug; you use it and then move on to something else. It wasn't intended to be used every day.

Take it from me: it's easy to put someone on a PPI, but it's a devil to get them off.

The second-biggest problem with PPIs is that they can reduce the effectiveness of other drugs and, in some cases, render them totally ineffective.

Take clopidogrel (Plavix), for example, an anticoagulant that's used to prevent strokes and heart attacks in patients at risk for these problems — typically those who've had stents surgically inserted to treat narrowed or weakened arteries in their bodies. Because PPIs shut down the enzymes in the liver that metabolize the Plavix, patients taking them often don't get any benefit from the anticoagulant at all and thus are at a higher risk for heart attack or stroke.

In 2009 the Food and Drug Administration warned that PPIs should not be used at the same time as Plavix, even if the drugs are taken many hours apart, because they can make the anticoagulant dangerously less effective.

In my daily practice, I can see that doctors often prescribe PPIs recklessly, as they're not aware of how many adverse interactions with other drugs they can trigger and how they pave the way for changes in drug metabolism that can harm the patients they're treating.

PPIs interfere with any drugs or nutrients that need an acid media to be absorbed, and the list of those medications and supplements is a long one indeed. It includes any drug in extended-release form as well as calcium and iron. Whenever a patient comes to me with anemia, I immediately look to see if a prescription PPI is on board. If not, I ask the patient if he or she is taking over-the-counter versions of the drug. With anemia, a proton pump inhibitor is nearly always the culprit, or at least a major contributing factor.

If a doctor prescribes a PPI along with one or more drugs that have a narrow therapeutic window (where the dose needed to be effective is close to a dose that could be toxic), the patient quickly gets into all kinds of problems as his or her blood chemistry starts changing.

In fact, PPIs can interfere with hundreds and hundreds of medications in this way.

So that you can picture the complexities and potential problems, here's just a short list of medications that should not be used at the same time as PPIs:

- H_2 blockers, including Tagamet, Pepcid, Axid, and Zantac
- any extended-release medication, such as metoprolol (Toprol XL), tolterodine (Detrol LA), and diltiazem (Cardizem CD), to name just a few
- calcium carbonate supplements (Adcal, Cacit, Calcichew, Caltrate, OsCal, etc.)
- iron salts (Albafort, Femiron, Feosol, and so on)
- cefpodoxime (Vantin)
- cefuroxime (Ceftin)
- citalopram (Celexa)
- clarithromycin (Biaxin)
- clopidogrel (Plavix)
- diazepam (Valium)
- digoxin (Lanoxin)
- escitalopram (Lexapro)
- fluconazole (Diflucan)
- itraconazole (Sporanox)
- ketoconazole (Feoris, Nizoral)
- methotrexate (Rheumatrex, Trexall)
- naproxen (Aleve)
- olanzapine (Zyprexa)

- penicillins
- phenytoins (Diphen, Dilantin, Pheny-tek)
- posaconazole (Noxafil)
- tacrolimus (Prograf)
- warfarin (Coumadin)

The other huge problem with proton pump inhibitors — the one I've saved for last — is that, for most patients with nonerosive forms of GERD, they don't really work.

"The failure of PPIs to resolve GERD symptoms has become the most commonly seen patient scenario in gastroenterology practices," observed an article published in 2009 in *Gut,* a leading international journal of gastroenterology. An analysis of GERD patients on a daily dose of a PPI, published in another gastroenterology journal in 2003, found that 25 percent to 40 percent continued to have symptoms.

I hope that this is enough to deter you from using a proton pump inhibitor, but if you remain unpersuaded, here are some other facts to consider:

PPIs increase your risk for bone loss and osteoporotic fractures. In 2010 the FDA investigated the need for label warnings on PPIs about the possibility of fracture risk, saying that the drugs may interfere with the ability of the digestive tract to absorb calcium, and in 2011 it issued a safety update, saying that patients who take higher-dose prescription PPIs or who take prescription PPIs for more than a year may face a greater risk for fractures.

Although no one knows exactly why or how PPIs increase fracture risk — there's a dearth of reliable data in this area — some researchers have suggested that these drugs may reduce bone resorption by inhibiting the proton pumps in osteoclasts, the cells that nibble at and break down bone.

The strongest evidence that PPIs increase fracture risk comes from the Nurses' Health Study, which is widely considered to be the most definitive long-term epidemiological (population-based) study ever conducted on the health of older women. The study, established in 1976, has followed more than 120,000 female registered nurses to assess risk factors for major chronic diseases.

A 2011 evaluation of data from the Nurses' Health Study shows that postmenopausal women in the study group using PPIs were at significantly higher risk of hip fractures than those not taking PPIs, and that the risk climbed with the duration of treatment: to 36 percent after two years, to 42 percent after four years, and to 54 percent after six years or longer. When proton pump inhibitors were discontinued, the analysis showed, the risk declined within two years to around 10 percent — a dramatic difference.

(Another detail of interest: in 2000, 7 percent of the nurses participating in the study reported that they were using PPIs; by 2008, that number had climbed to 19 percent.)

Whenever a patient comes to me complaining of bone pain, I immediately look to see if a PPI could be the culprit. Because they prevent the body from absorbing calcium in the stomach, the body is going to start searching for it elsewhere. And if it can't find the calcium it needs in the stomach, it's going to start pulling it out of the bones.

PPIs increase your risk of hypomagnesemia, an abnormally low level of magnesium in the blood. Hypomagnesemia can lead to disturbances in nearly every organ system and cause potentially fatal complications, including abnormally rapid heartbeats, coronary vasospasms (a form of angina, or chest pain, caused when the coronary artery spasms), and sudden death.

The FDA sounded this warning in the safety alert for prescription PPIs that it issued in 2011, noting that hypomagnesemia is probably underrecognized and underreported. The agency's alert pointed out that low serum magnesium levels can cause other serious problems such as muscle spasms and seizures. It further recommended that doctors check a patient's serum magnesium level before prescribing a PPI as well as do periodic follow-ups with patients who take PPIs for prolonged periods or who take them with digoxin (Lanoxin), a drug used to treat heart failure and abnormal heart rhythms, or drugs such as diuretics that can also cause hypomagnesemia. In my experience, these checks are never done.

PPIs may increase your risk of adenocarcinoma, a lethal form of esophageal cancer. A study by a team of researchers at the University of Pittsburgh School of Medicine, published in 2001 in the journal *Archives of Surgery,* found that patients using PPIs were much less likely to undergo endoscopic screening that could detect Barrett's esophagus, a precursor to adenocarcinoma — the fastest-growing cancer in the Western world. "We are learning that the chronic and long-term use of PPIs may not be entirely without consequences," one of the study's authors explained, "and may lead to more insidious problems or cause one to be asymptomatic in the face of continued esophageal injury from GERD." In short, PPIs can mask the symptoms of Barrett's esophagus, dramatically increasing the chances that it will transform, undetected, into cancer.

PPIs increase the risk for serious infections, such as *C. difficile* and pneumonia. Multiple studies show that PPI therapy is associated with increases in the incidence of *C. difficile* — the "superbug" that causes severe and often fatal diarrhea. Acid-suppressing drugs like proton pump inhibitors create a more favorable environment in the stomach for the spores of the *C. difficile* bacteria to germinate. The spores have a heyday in a basic pH environment, which is what the gut becomes with prolonged PPI use.

C. difficile infections are extremely contagious. They spread when the spores, which can survive outside of the human body for very long periods of time, are accidentally ingested by patients in hospitals, nursing homes, and similar facilities. One study of hospital-acquired *C. difficile* cases found that 64 percent of the patients were on a PPI when the infection developed. The report's authors could find no valid indication for PPI therapy in 63 percent of the cases — a finding, as explained later, that most certainly has to do with hospital procedures aimed at maximizing Medicare reimbursements. Almost every hospital in the nation has a standing order to put patients on PPIs as soon as they are admitted, because the government will not pay for hospital services if the patient develops a stress ulcer while in the hospital.

PPI use is a significant risk factor for nursing home residents. A study published in the *Journal of the American Medical Directors Association* found that about 60 percent of nursing home residents with *C. difficile*-associated disease were taking proton pump inhibitors, versus 32 percent of those not taking PPIs. What so often happens is that patients are discharged from the hospital still on the PPI therapy that was inappropriately initiated there, and they go directly to the nursing home, where the therapy is never stopped.

Multiple studies have also linked PPI use

to higher rates of pneumonia, including pneumonia acquired in hospitals. This is almost certainly because gastric acid is the body's first line of defense against infection. Most bacteria can't survive at the stomach's normal pH level, but once the pH level is pushed to basic by PPI therapy, you very quickly develop bacterial overgrowth. Then, when you aspirate stomach contents, drawing them into the lower respiratory tract (which includes the windpipe), you get pneumonia.

PPIs increase your risk of vitamin B_{12} deficiency. The older you are, the greater your risk of vitamin B_{12} deficiency, and PPIs can make things much worse. Vitamin B_{12} is bound to proteins in foods such as meat, fish, poultry, eggs, and dairy products; when those foods reach the stomach, acids and enzymes break down the proteins and release the B_{12} for the body to use. PPIs, by suppressing stomach acids, make it more difficult for the body to extract vitamin B_{12} from the foods you eat. This is an especially serious problem for older people because they lack intrinsic factor (IF), the essential enzyme needed to absorb vitamin B_{12}, and the PPI therapy makes it impossible for them to get any B_{12}. The vitamin B_{12}

deficiency that results causes impaired cognition, dementia, poor muscle tone, and many other neuromuscular problems.

Older adults with vitamin B_{12} deficiency are more likely to suffer from depression (according to a study published in 2011 in the *American Journal of Clinical Nutrition*) and sleep disturbances.

PPIs, when taken to reduce the chances of developing ulcers from NSAID therapy, may simply shift the damage to the small intestine. PPIs are frequently prescribed at the same time as nonsteroidal anti-inflammatory medications to reduce NSAID-induced GI bleeding and other gastroduodenal injuries. But a study by scientists at the Farncombe Family Digestive Health Research Institute at McMaster University in Canada, published in 2011 in the journal *Gastroenterology,* found that PPIs may actually be aggravating damage elsewhere. "These drugs appear to be shifting the damage from the stomach to the small intestine, where the ulcers may be more dangerous and more difficult to treat," John Wallace, MD, the institute's director, explained.

Because most doctors aren't aware of the

serious risks associated with proton pump inhibitors, the nation is awash in unnecessary prescriptions for these dangerous drugs. They're so dangerous, as I see it, that they shouldn't even be available in nonprescription form, and I think it's really just a matter of time until PPIs are no longer available over the counter.

Something like 90 percent of the patients who come through my office door are on a PPI at the time of our initial consultation. Many of them were put on a PPI in the hospital and were never taken off afterward. Nearly always this has to do with the fact that Medicare won't pay a claim if a patient develops a stress ulcer while in the hospital. The crazy thing about this is that study after study has shown that PPI therapy does not prevent stress ulcers. And so putting the patient on the PPI has nothing to do with his or her needs — that is, it's not related to any medical diagnosis — but with the hospital's desire to see to it that all of its claims are processed without a hitch.

As it turns out, this practice is based spuriously on studies of critically ill patients in intensive care units, not on non-ICU patients. The most recent and most comprehensive research study in this area, published in the *Archives of Internal Medicine* in

2011, found that 770 patients need to be treated with PPIs to prevent 1 hospital-acquired GI bleed and that 834 patients need to be treated to prevent 1 clinically significant GI bleed. That study, carried out by four doctors affiliated with Beth Israel Deaconness Medical Center, a teaching hospital of Harvard Medical School, should have been enough to end this wasteful and dangerous practice. But the willy-nilly use of PPIs in hospitals goes on. As I see it, it all has to do with drug company profits, as the manufacturers of PPIs practically give them to the hospital so as to be the only such drug on the formulary, knowing that their drug will follow patients after they are discharged from the hospital. And when those patients end up in nursing homes, assisted living homes, or back in their own homes, they'll still be on drugs that they never needed in the first place.

But what if it's your doctor who's suggesting the PPI?

If you're one of the many Americans who experience heartburn each day — and up to fifteen million Americans are said to be in this category — there are alternatives to PPIs that are far, far safer and nearly always are more effective. These alternatives are built around changing problematic diet and lifestyle habits, not taking a drug every day to compensate for them.

Before the new classes of acid-supressing drugs were invented, people kept their diets and lifestyles in check so as to avoid the kinds of problems that today send them to the doctor or drugstore in search of a medication that will help. They ate dinner earlier (leaving more time to digest their food), for example, and went to bed later, for example, and as a rule, they didn't eat the spicy foods they eat today. And they had some safe remedies — such as drinking a glass of cultured buttermilk — that many doctors today wrongly dismiss as ineffectual.

If you're bothered by heartburn or occasional acid reflux, here's the initial to-do list I'd give you, presented here in ultrashort form:

- If you smoke, quit.
- If you're overweight, shed some of your excess poundage.
- Avoid spicy, fatty, or fried foods, along with garlic, onions, citrus fruits, and any other foods that seem to trigger heartburn, such as tomato-based products.
- Avoid caffeine and chocolate.

- Avoid carbonated drinks and citrus juices.
- Limit your consumption of alcohol to no more than two ounces a day.
- Eat small meals.
- Eat more fiber.
- Consume nonfat or low-fat yogurt or cultured buttermilk throughout the day, every day, and always at bedtime.
- Chew sugar-free gum after meals. It increases peristalsis, the symmetrical contraction and relaxation of stomach muscles, and helps move acid through the gut.
- Don't wear tight belts or clothing that's tight around the waist.
- Don't bend over or exercise immediately after eating.
- Eat at least three hours before your bedtime, and eat even earlier if you can.
- Elevate the head of your bed.

If these suggested changes seem too overwhelming, you may want to focus on the two interventions that studies show to be most effective: losing some weight and raising the head of your bed. If you still need relief, use one of the newer over-the-counter H_2 blockers such as Zantac for relief — but only on an occasional basis and in a dose of no more than 75 milligrams a day.

You may also want to consider trying a melatonin supplement. Melatonin, a natural hormone that can be produced synthetically, helps to regulate the body's circadian rhythm (our twenty-four-hour internal "clock") and is also a powerful antioxidant. One study, published in the *Journal of Pineal Research* in 2006, compared 176 patients taking melatonin and some additional nutrients (tryptophan, vitamins B_6 and B_{12}, the amino acid methionine, betaine, and folic acid) with 175 patients on a 20-milligram daily dose of Prilosec. The results were remarkable.

After seven days, 90 percent of the patients taking the melatonin and nutrients were free of heartburn or reflux symptoms; after forty days, 100 percent were symptom free, compared with 66 percent of the patients taking Prilosec. The patients in the latter group who still reported symptoms were then given the melatonin-nutrients combination for forty days. At the end of this period, all of these PPI "nonresponders" were free of heartburn or reflux symptoms.

I mention this study not so much as an endorsement of melatonin therapy but to suggest that sometimes alternative approaches are worth trying, especially in older patients. The use of yogurt and buttermilk, for example, may seem old-fashioned to some, but it works extremely well in very old patients and typically produces the desired outcome without turning their body chemistry upside down.

What if your doctor insists that you need to stay on a proton pump inhibitor? When my patients find themselves in this position, I give them a copy of an editorial published by the journal *Gastroenterology* in 2009. Written by two leading experts on the adverse effects of PPIs — Kenneth E. L. McColl, MD, and Derek Gillen, MD, both of the Division of Cardiovascular and Medical Sciences at the University of Glasgow, in Scotland — the editorial, "Evidence That Proton-Pump Inhibitor Therapy Induces the Symptoms It Is Used to Treat," pointed to a study in the journal suggesting that PPIs may cause or aggravate the disease process they are used to treat. Drs. McColl and Gillen write:

[A] substantial proportion, if not majority, of patients now prescribed proton pump inhibitor therapy do not have acid-related symptoms and therefore have no true indication for such therapy. The current finding that these drugs induce symptoms means that such liberal [mis-] prescribing is likely to be creating the disease the drugs are designed to treat and causing patients with no previous need for such therapy to require intermittent or long-term treatment. It is likely also that treatment of mild reflux symptoms with such therapy may aggravate the underlying disease and lead to an increased requirement for long-term therapy.

How long will it take most doctors who prescribe PPIs to reach the same sensible conclusion? I hope it won't be too long, but experience tells me not to hold my breath.

For some time now, I've been working with an eighty-four-year-old patient who came to me on 80 milligrams of Nexium a day. He's been on this very high dose for more than five years. He's in so much bone pain that his list of opiate analgesic drugs is long — another problem that needs to be resolved. After three months of tapering the PPI therapy, I have him down to 60 milligrams daily. As you can see, it's an extremely slow process. But the PPI problem has to be resolved before any of his other problems can be addressed, because with the Nexium-induced liver-isozyme shutdown, other changes in his drug therapy are impossible. At this point, I can only hope that he lives long enough for us to correct this horrible mistake and allow him to be free from pain once again.

STATIN ROULETTE:
DRUGS OF LAST RESORT

More than thirty million Americans, by one estimate, take statin drugs. Statins are prescribed mostly to lower LDL ("bad") cholesterol; they include atorvastatin (Lipitor), pravastatin (Pravachol), rosuvastatin (Crestor), and simvastatin (Zocor). Statins are the best-selling class of drugs in the United States, and atorvastatin is the best-selling prescription drug in history.

If you're sixty-five or older, the odds are pretty good that you're taking a statin — especially if you're a man. According to the most recent data from the National Center for Health Statistics, 50 percent of all men ages sixty-five to seventy-four, and 45 percent of all men seventy-five and older, take statins; so do 36 percent of women age sixty-five to seventy-four, and 39 percent of women seventy-five and older.

Statins have been certified as safe by the American College of Cardiology, the American Heart Association, and the National Heart, Lung, and Blood Institute, among other organizations.

Over the years I've heard many internists say that everybody over the age of forty should be on a statin drug. And then, of course, there's the idea that statins are so effective and so safe that they ought to be added to the water supply, a misguided notion that may have been launched in 2004 by John Reckless, MD, a physician and endocrinologist in Bath, England, whose official biography notes that he has "a national reputation in the management of lipid disorders in the general population."

At the annual meeting of Heart UK (the British organization that bills itself as "the cholesterol charity"), the BBC reported at the time, Dr. Reckless remarked that "maybe people should be able to have their statin, perhaps if not in their drinking water, with their drinking water."

Not me. In the years since statins came into widespread use, I've come to believe that they're among the most ineffective and dangerous drugs on the market, largely because the doctors who prescribe them haven't done their homework, relying instead on information supplied by the manufacturers of statins and the studies they've underwritten. I stop these drugs on all the older patients I see because they are invariably at the root of nearly all their problems.

Robert Lemmon, MD, a family doctor in Seneca, South Carolina, who's written a series of online monographs on what he calls "overrated medicines" (statins among them), has explained from personal experience how physicians come to toe the pharmaceutical industry's line so easily. Here's how Dr. Lemmon put it:

> I, like most primary care physicians, had the "statins are good, add them to the drinking water" mentality drilled into my head at lectures paid for by Big Pharma. Eloquent cardiologists with rapier wit expounded on the studies while I dined on filet mignon and pinot noir. I left the lectures after hearing impressive risk reduction numbers like 33 percent for cardiovascular death and 22 percent for all-cause death . . . Like most family physicians (and other specialists, I suspect), I never read the actual studies. I just accepted what the speakers paid for by Big Pharma told me.

Statins lower the levels of LDL (low-density

lipoprotein) cholesterol in the body by interfering with the liver's ability to produce it. The liver produces about 75 percent of the cholesterol that circulates in our blood; the rest comes from the food we eat.

Elevated LDL levels are worrisome from a medical standpoint because they can lead to the formation of deposits called plaques within the walls of the coronary arteries (the vessels that carry oxygen-rich blood to the heart muscle); as the plaques accumulate, they may bulge into the arteries and begin interfering with the blood flow. If one of the plaques ruptures, the sudden blood clot that forms over the rupture can lead to a heart attack or stroke.

It's important to remember that you can have high cholesterol without having coronary artery disease (atherosclerosis), a condition that used to be commonly known as "hardening of the arteries." Some of this has to do with how much HDL ("good") cholesterol you have in your body. The higher your HDL (high-density lipoprotein) levels, the better off you are. If your HDL is above 45, then high LDL is not that important to treat.

HDL cholesterol circulates through the bloodstream, vacuuming up the bad LDL cholesterol and transporting it to the liver, where it can be reprocessed just as nature intended. (Our internal recycling systems were designed, of course, well before such artery-clogging inventions as triple cheeseburgers and deep-fried Twinkies came along.)

The therapeutic goal, in my judgment, should always be to keep the two cholesterol levels — good HDL and bad LDL — in balance and to deal at the same time with other risk factors, such as obesity and tobacco use, that can push a person into heart disease.

It's also important to recognize that older people can have high levels of an essential amino acid called homocysteine in their blood, and that this in itself can cause elevated LDL levels. Instead of attacking the problem with statins, all that may be needed is to use vitamin-B-complex therapy (a combination of folic acid, vitamin B_6, and vitamin B_{12}) — and thus the body's own chemistry — to lower the homocysteine levels.

If you're taking a statin now, your doctor, in prescribing the drug, has probably placed you in one of two treatment categories. The first is primary prevention. In this case, you probably have high cholesterol but no known coronary artery disease; your doctor's assumption is that the statin will help prevent you from developing heart disease or having a heart attack. The other is secondary prevention. In this case, you have probably been diagnosed with coronary artery disease and may even have had one or more heart attacks; your doctor's assumption is that the statin will help prevent or at least reduce your risk of heart attack.

Most of the patients I see for the first time, both in my office and in nursing homes, are on statins. Nearly always, I find that the statins are causing major problems that have gone unrecognized as drug effects. And nearly always, I wonder why they were prescribed in the first place. If you don't have hardening of the arteries by the time you're seventy or eighty, you most likely never will, and if you do have this problem, it's too late for a statin drug to help you.

Unfortunately, too many doctors fall into the filet-mignon-and-pinot-noir trap that Dr. Lemmon describes and, as a consequence, look to the drug manufacturers as their primary source of information. This virtually guarantees that they will prescribe the drugs more often than they should and that the benefits of the drugs will nearly always seem to outweigh their risks dramatically.

That's why I feel that a back-to-basics approach is so helpful with patients. And for statins, here are the basics:

Despite what you've been told, statins may not reduce your risk of death. If you've been prescribed a statin because you fall into the primary-prevention category described above (and 75 percent of all people who take statins do), you'd do well to question whether you really need to be taking the drug and whether it might be doing more harm than good. That's especially important if you're older or if you've been taking a statin for several years or more.

A comprehensive review of previous studies published in 2011 by the Cochrane Collaboration, a well-respected nonprofit research organization, found no "strong evidence" that statins reduce deaths from coronary heart disease among patients who have not suffered a heart attack or other cardiovascular event in the past. The Cochrane authors, reviewing data from fourteen studies involving 34,272 patients, concluded that 1,000 patients in that category have to be treated for one year to prevent one death.

A similar review of statin studies published

in the *Archives of Internal Medicine* in 2010 reached a similar conclusion. "[T]here is little evidence that statins reduce the risk of dying from any cause in individuals without heart disease," the authors wrote.

Lee A. Green, MD, a professor in the Department of Family Medicine at the University of Michigan, wrote in an accompanying commentary, "The meta-analysis makes it clear that in the short term, for true primary prevention, the benefit, if any, is very small. In the long term, we really must admit that we do not know."

Statins can destroy your muscles. The most common unwanted effects of statins involve the muscles. When I see an older patient who complains of muscle pain, fatigue, and weakness, I know from experience that a statin drug is the most likely culprit. In my judgment, muscle-related adverse effects are much more prevalent than the literature suggests because they often go undiagnosed or misdiagnosed.

Muscle weakness and severe muscle aches throughout the body can be symptoms of statin-induced rhabdomyolysis, a rapid breakdown of skeletal muscle that causes muscle fibers to be released into the bloodstream. The fibers are harmful to the kidneys and frequently result in severe kidney damage and even kidney failure. The higher the dose of statins, the higher the risk of rhabdomyolysis.

The use of certain other drugs in combination with statins — fibric acid derivatives, or fibrates, for example, which are typically prescribed to lower blood triglyceride levels — also increases the risk of rhabdomyolysis. (This class of medications includes bezafibrate [Bezalip], ciprofibrate [Modalim], gemfibrozil [Lopid], and fenofibrate [TriCor].) The package insert for Pravachol, for example, makes clear that if you take the drug with a fibrate, "you may have an increased risk for serious reactions, including serious muscle problems."

Because either drug can cause muscle problems on its own, the combined use of the drugs exponentially increases the risks of such adverse effects. One Harvard study, for example, found that the combination of a statin and a fibrate multiplies the risk of muscle damage more than sixfold.

Although it's been known for many years that statins and fibrates generally should not be used together, I see patients on both types of drugs with frightening frequency.

The Food and Drug Administration

warned doctors in June 2011 that the use of simvastatin (Zocor, Vytorin) in 80-milligram doses should be avoided because of the risk of muscle damage.

One of the big issues is that statin-induced muscle problems often don't go away when the drug is discontinued. A study of statin-induced myopathies (muscle diseases) published in the journal *Muscle & Nerve* in 2006 found that "variable persistent symptoms occurred in 68 percent of patients despite cessation of therapy."

Statins can cause serious cognitive problems. These are second only to muscle problems among the adverse effects reported by patients taking statins.

A study published in 2004 by Matthew F. Muldoon, MD, and his colleagues at the University of Pittsburgh School of Medicine found the use of statins to be associated with a variety of cognitive problems. They examined 283 patients with high cholesterol who were treated over a six-month trial with simvastatin in 10- and 40-milligram doses or with placebo, giving them cognitive function tests before and after. The researchers found that the patients on statins, as a group, showed major declines in performance on tests assessing attention, memory, and overall mental efficiency. The results of a 2001 study had reported similar findings for another statin drug, lovastatin (Mevacor).

A study based on patient surveys that was published in the journal *Pharmacotherapy* in 2009 found that 75 percent of the subjects "experienced cognitive ADRs [adverse drug reactions] determined to be probably or definitely related to statin therapy," and that 90 percent of the patients who stopped statin therapy reported improvements in cognition, sometimes within days. According to the study, some patients even reported having a diagnosis of dementia or Alzheimer's disease reversed after they had stopped taking statins.

Occasionally you even run across psychiatrists who've seen much the same thing. Emily Deans, MD, a clinical instructor in psychiatry at Harvard Medical School and a practicing psychiatrist in the Boston area, recently wrote on KevinMD.com, a Web site of physician commentaries, "I've had three patients with increased paranoia or psychosis that began with starting the statin and resolved with removing the statin. Numerous other 'foggy brains' and difficult-to-treat depressions became much simpler once the statin was removed."

251

Statins may increase your risk of developing diabetes. Researchers at Glasgow University in Scotland analyzed thirteen clinical trials of statin drugs from 1994 to 2009 involving more than 91,000 patients. They concluded that statin use is associated with a "slightly increased" risk of developing type 2 diabetes. Similarly, an analysis of statin studies that was published in the *Journal of the American Medical Association* in 2011 found that people who were treated with high doses of statins were more likely to develop diabetes than those treated with moderate doses.

If you've had a hemorrhagic stroke, taking statins may increase your risk of having another one. Many patients at risk of hemorrhagic stroke — the type of stroke that occurs when a blood vessel in the brain bursts or breaks — are prescribed statins. But a team of researchers from Massachusetts General Hospital and Harvard Medical School reported in the *Archives of Neurology* in 2011 that using statins in such patients actually increased their risk of a second hemorrhagic stroke by up to 22 percent, offsetting any possible cardiovascular benefits. "[T]he risk of statin therapy," an accompanying editorial noted, "likely outweighs any potential benefit in patients with (at least recent) brain hemorrhage and should generally be avoided."

Statins can interfere with your ability to metabolize other drugs. Some of the most widely prescribed statins are metabolized by a liver enzyme known as CYP3A4. It has been estimated that half of all prescription drugs are metabolized by CYP3A4. As a result, drugs that interfere with the CYP3A4 pathway — or that merely compete within it — can lead to a wide variety of adverse drug reactions, the buildup of drugs within the liver to toxic levels, and the lessening of intended pharmacological effects.

The older you are, the more dangerous statin drugs may be. Nearly every day, I see elderly patients who have been taking statin drugs for many years. Although there is next to no evidence that hypercholesterolemia — high blood cholesterol levels — is a risk factor in this age group, most doctors simply assume that it is and write a prescription for a statin without so much as a second thought.

But there's solid evidence that the indiscriminate prescribing of statins to very old people is ill advised, according to a team of Danish researchers who reviewed observational studies and randomized clinical trials of statin use in that age group. Writing in the journal *Age and Ageing* in 2010, they concluded, "There is not sufficient data to recommend anything regarding initiation or continuation of lipid-lowering treatment for the population aged 80+, with known cardiovascular disease (CVD), and it is even possible that statins may increase all-cause mortality in this group of elderly individuals without CVD."

Doctors often fail to recognize the side effects of statin drugs and prescribe additional drugs to treat problems that could be resolved simply by withdrawing the statins. Whenever I see patients who've been diagnosed with restless leg syndrome (RLS), a neurological disorder that causes all kinds of discomfort and sleeping problems, I've learned to check immediately to see if there's a statin on board. There nearly always is. Typically, the patient has complained to her doctor of RLS-like symptoms — persistent aches, cramps, and jittery feelings in her legs and other limbs — and the doctor has responded with a prescription for the dopamine agonist ropinirole (Requip) or another drug. Thus the prescription cascade begins.

Other telltale signs of statin toxicity include pain in the muscles and joints; stomach pain (which I tend to believe results from damage to the muscles in the stomach and diaphragm); trouble swallowing (also a muscle problem); balance problems; difficulties standing and climbing steps; and elevated liver enzymes.

Doctors often dismiss even the possibility that the statin drugs they've prescribed could be causing the adverse effects their patients complain about, even when there is ample evidence of causality. A study published in the journal *Drug Safety* in 2007 looked at the cases of 650 adults on statins who had muscle pain, cognitive impairment, or other recognized symptoms of statin toxicity. The study reported that 87 percent of the patients talked with their doctors about whether these symptoms could be related to their use of statins, and that the vast majority of the discussions were initiated by the patients, not their physicians. More often than not, the doctors rejected the notion that the statins might have any relationship at all to the symptoms.

Not long ago, one of the nursing homes at which I work admitted an eighty-seven-year-old woman who, in addition to a statin, had been prescribed a dopamine agonist for restless leg syndrome, an antiepileptic for neuropathic pain, an antipsychotic for hallucinations, and a combination L-dopa-carbidopa drug for tremors. I knew that once the statin was stopped, all the other problems would likely go away. That's exactly what happened, as it turned out, and within thirty days, she was discharged home with her daughter. At that point, she was taking only a single pill: a multi-vitamin.

I first met John Harkness on September 22, 2009. He'd driven down from Jackson, Georgia, which is about twenty miles east of Griffin, for an initial consultation. I later recorded my observations as follows:

This sixty-three-year-old white male presents with multiple drugs; swelling in his legs; dermatitis on his legs; neuropathy in his extremities; leg, back, and muscle pain; extreme anxiety and depression; and confusion that his doctor cannot diagnose or define. Being frustrated and hurting has resulted in a very high degree of anxiety and depression that was obvious at the start of our interview.

Assessment with the short Geriatric Depression Scale produced a value of 13, which indicates an immediate need for therapeutic intervention. It is hard to understand why, in numerous visits, the physician hasn't picked up on his extreme depression and initiated some type of treatment. Reviewing his medications shows many problem areas that result in the current symptoms he is experiencing.

In reviewing Mr. Harkness's morning and evening blood pressure readings and pulse values, I could see that an improvement in his diastolic blood pressure was needed. It was also a sign that the ACE inhibitor he'd been prescribed (benazepril; brand name, Lotensin) wasn't really working and was probably the cause of the swelling in his legs, rash, and neuropathy.

Making things worse, the benazepril had been prescribed along with the statin drug Lipitor as well as colchicine (Colcrys), a plant-derived drug used to treat acute attacks of gout. We know from studies that the concomitant use of these drugs can lead to myotoxicity, which is basically a poisoning of the muscles. This condition begins with muscle pain and weakness and progresses to rhabdomyolysis.

Rhabdomyolysis is often accompanied by renal dysfunction and sometimes by renal failure and death. An assortment of toxicities involving the heart, pancreas, liver, bone marrow, and respiratory and central nervous systems has also been reported.

I could tell from calculating Mr. Harkness's creatinine clearance (74 cc/min) that he had enough renal impairment to put him at high risk for these muscle problems. His angioedema (swelling beneath the skin) was another adverse effect associated with the use of the drugs.

My basic recommendations were to discontinue the colchicine and replace it with the antigout medication allopurinol (Zyloprim); discontinue the benazepril, which wasn't working, and replace it with a benzothiazepine calcium channel blocker (diltiazem CD), which older patients can metabolize effectively; and discontinue the Lipitor and instead try to control his lipids with a combination of vitamin B_{12} injections, folic acid, and vitamin B_6.

I explained to Mr. Harkness that Lipitor, like all of the statin drugs, can have adverse effects on the skeletal muscles, which are the muscles that allow the body to move. A study published in 2008 found that statin drugs caused fatigue, muscle cramping, and potential myopathy, and, in 9 percent of the patients studied, statin-related pain.

When I saw Mr. Harkness for a follow-up visit the next month, the swelling in his legs was completely gone. He told me that the feeling was coming back into his body and that he was sleeping through the night, something that he hadn't done in years.

His morning blood pressure readings were still higher than they should have been, but with some adjustment, we brought his diastolic values in line by switching to two doses a day of the diltiazem CD. There were also improvements in his lipids profile (a reduction of about 30 points in his LDL and about 35 points in his cholesterol, and an increase of 20 points in his HDL, along with a reduction in his triglycerides, a type of fat in the blood).

By the following spring, Mr. Harkness's risk of developing "hard" coronary heart disease, as measured by the Framingham Heart Study risk assessment tool, had dropped from 20 percent to 16 percent, which is very favorable for his age group.

That's the story from my point of view. I

thought you'd also be interested in hearing the story from his perspective, exactly as he posted it one day on the AARP Web site in the "Comments" field below a story about my work. This is pretty much just as Mr. Harkness wrote it:

After spending a week in the local hospital and having been poked, prodded, tested, and injected, I was sent home with a diagnosis of: "Sometimes as we age, things happen that appear to have no cause or cure . . . This is something you will have to learn to live with." (My whole body was swollen to the point that I could not walk. Both legs were swollen to the point of rupture and were oozing fluid. I couldn't breathe, causing my blood oxygen level to be in the sixties.)

I had heard about Dr. Neel several years prior, and looked up his number and called. He gave me a quick appointment. I waddled into his office and was ushered into his interview room. One quick look at my legs, and he gave a diagnosis promptly: rhabdomyolysis, brought on by a reaction to the prescription for Lipitor. Within 24 hours of stopping the Lipitor, the swelling was gone.

Dr. Neel, upon request, suggested a

local doctor who did not object to suggestions to help his patients. Between the two of them, I was given a new regimen of prescription drugs and over-the-counter products to replace the sackful of prescriptions I had been on for years. Dr. Neel and my new doctor turned my miserable life around and put me on the road to recovery. The bloodwork and detailed attention paid me saved my life. I also had a thyroid that didn't work, a prostate that was malfunctioning, a bad gene that left me subject to all sorts of old-age problems, a pancreatic proclivity for overproduction of insulin, and a staggering amount of weight gain. These two men working together addressed each health issue individually and corrected these problems one at a time.

To date, I have lost 83 pounds and continue to lose. I can walk easily without pain and have resumed my old activities of which I was deprived for three years. I feel good, and look forward to spending time with my grandchildren for years to come. I credit Dr. Armon Neel with saving my life!!!

John Harkness's story isn't an aberration. It's actually more in the nature of the rule, in fact, than the exception.

Not long ago, a close friend asked me if I'd be willing to help a colleague whose eighty-five-year-old father was experiencing seemingly insurmountable medical problems. He'd been hospitalized several times in the past six months for cardiovascular events and infections, and he'd emerged from the most recent hospitalization with a urinary catheter (he'd previously been diagnosed with an enlarged prostate gland) and an inability to get around on his own, even with a walker. (He'd also been diagnosed previously with an unspecified "movement disorder.") The man's son had confided in my friend that he feared his father might not live to see his next birthday.

The son, with the help of his sister, faxed me a list of the medications his father was taking along with some lab results that I had requested. There was the statin Lipitor, which he seemed to have been taking longer than any of the other drugs. There was tamsulosin (Flomax), an alpha-blocker that's used to treat benign prostatic hyperplasia (BPH). There was a very high dose of Stalevo, a combination drug used to treat the symptoms of Parkinson's disease that contains carbidopa, levodopa, and entacapone. There were more than a half dozen other drugs on top of these, but as I looked over the list and the labs, I kept coming back to the Lipitor. There was a good chance, it seemed to me, that it was the source of most of his problems.

The family managed to talk the doctors into discontinuing the Lipitor immediately and gradually stepping down the Stalevo with the goal of withdrawing it too. The motion-disorder specialist who'd prescribed the Stalevo apparently warned the family that there was a danger the patient would choke to death on discontinuing the drug, but they decided that it was a risk worth taking.

In just about ten days, the father's condition began improving dramatically. The catheter was removed, never to come back. He was soon able to get out of bed on his own, and then to get around again with the walker, and he began setting new distance records on almost a daily basis. His voice, which had been reduced to a raspy whisper, returned full throttle. He began telling his wife that his head felt clear for the first time, and his daughter was amazed to see him laughing, cracking jokes, and talking about playing bridge again for the first time in more than a year. And then, completing his miraculous turnaround, he was discharged from the nursing facility to return to the apartment he'd shared with his wife in the same community.

He's not worried these days about high cholesterol. Nor is he worried about his "motion disorder," which seems to have vanished with the discontinuation of the drugs. What's more, he's actually putting back on some of the weight he'd lost, as his appetite returned to normal and he found it far easier — not more difficult — to swallow. And he's awake for most of the day, even without the methylphenidate (Ritalin) they'd had him on in an effort to counteract the sedating effects of all the anticholinergic drugs they'd been giving him.

His family thought this all to be a miracle, but I knew it to be, really, anything but that. Every now and then I read a first-person account by someone I've never met that tells me I'm not alone in my thinking. Consider, for example, the story of Katherine Farady, MD, a dermatologist in Austin, Texas, as she posted it on a Web site read mostly by doctors:

At the age of 46, I started taking Lipitor for familial hypercholesterolemia. I was healthy. Within six months, I was suffering from cardiac arrhythmias, fatigue, colitis/chronic diarrhea, generalized anxiety and a major depression, as well as severe memory lapses. All these problems cost me thousands of dollars in physician visits and medications (at one count, I was taking seven different meds, besides the Lipitor). After two years of misery, I finally stopped the Lipitor on my own. The diarrhea and arrhythmias stopped within three weeks. Now, after two and a half years, I feel like I'm almost back to my baseline energy level.

The ironic thing is that I am a physician. I saw over eight different specialists during my illness and none of them (even me) suspected the statin as the cause of my ills. I have done a lot of research since then, and now know that there is no overall mortality benefit to taking statins for women, and no real benefit for primary prevention. Even the risk reduction for secondary prevention is rather small, given the cost of treatment (146 high-risk men in the WOSCOPS [West of Scotland Coronary Prevention Study] trial had to be treated with statins for five years to prevent one death).

I know this is an anecdotal story, but I have seen many patients in my dermatology practice who are on statins for no other reason than that their cholesterol is "a little high." Many of these patients are women, for whom no mortality benefit has ever been shown. And many of these patients are also on anti-depressants, or suffering from various other mysterious ailments. Makes you wonder. I also strongly believe that physicians who prescribe statins tend to dismiss patient complaints. I have seen it and experienced it myself. Every one of my side effects can be found in the PDR [*Physicians' Desk Reference*]. I was falling apart, yet my primary physician was happy because my cholesterol numbers looked good.

Anyone who's taking a statin drug, or who's being urged to take a statin drug, should read one or more of the studies that propelled them to blockbuster status. The West of Scotland Coronary Prevention Study that Dr. Farady mentions is a good place to start.

Before WOSCOPS was published in the *New England Journal of Medicine* in 1996, it had been postulated, but not proved, that lowering a patient's cholesterol levels could reduce the risk of cardiovascular disease as well as the risk of death from cardiovascular disease. WOSCOPS was hailed as the proof from the moment of its publication, and even today it is cited as the gold-standard evidence that statins save lives.

So let's take a close look.

The clinical trial examined 6,595 patients with very high cholesterol levels over nearly five years, with about half of them taking pravastatin and about half placebo. A good number of the patients had additional risk factors. Some 16 percent had high blood pressure, for example, and 44 percent were smokers. "When the effect of treatment with pravastatin on death from all cardiovascular causes was analyzed," the authors of the study reported, "a 32 percent reduction in risk was observed." The researchers also reported "a 22 percent reduction in the overall risk of death."

We have two ways of calculating reductions in risk. One, known as relative risk reduction, expresses the difference between two numbers as a percentage of one of the numbers. Let's assume, for a moment, that you have a 0.8 percent risk of dying in the next five years as a result of complications from high blood pressure. A new drug comes along that reduces your risk of dying to 0.4 percent. That's a relative risk reduction of 50 percent. If a doctor explains to you as he or she writes a prescription for the new wonder drug that it will cut your risk of dying from hypertension-related causes in half, it's true — as far as it goes. But the doctor is telling you nothing about how the drug affects your actual risk of dying.

The other measurement, known as absolute risk reduction, does just that. In this case, the absolute risk reduction is 0.4 percent — the difference between the starting risk of 0.8 percent and the modified risk (from taking the drug) of 0.4 percent.

Before we return to pravastatin, let's also look at a measure known as number needed to treat, or NNT. It's the number of patients you need to treat over a specified period to prevent one additional adverse outcome (heart attack, stroke, death, and so forth). In the case of our hypothetical hypertension drug, for example, the NNT is 250 (100/ 0.4), meaning that 250 patients would have to take the drug for five years to prevent 1 additional death from hypertension-related causes.

Keep in mind, too, that these various expressions of risk don't take into account any adverse events short of death, leading to all sorts of other questions. Would you take the drug for five years to avoid having a 1-in-250 chance of dying if it gave you a low-grade headache every day or gave you severe but non-life-threatening rashes?

But let's leave the realm of the hypothetical and return to Pravachol, the West of Scotland Coronary Prevention Study, and its authors' conclusion that use of the drug resulted in a "32 percent reduction in risk" of death from all cardiovascular causes and "a 22 percent reduction in the overall risk of death."

These results, expressed as relative risk reductions, certainly sound impressive, which is exactly what the authors of the study were aiming for. But if you look at the actual risk reductions, I think you'll agree that the results of the WOSCOPS trial were anything but impressive.

The absolute risk reductions from WOSCOPS can be calculated as 0.7 percent for death from cardiovascular causes over 4.9 years and 0.9 percent for death from all causes. In other words, 143 men have to take Pravachol for nearly five years to prevent 1 additional cardiovascular death, and 111 men have to take Pravachol for nearly five years to prevent 1 additional death from any cause.

If you read the study itself carefully, you may spot the most important sentence of all: "[I]t can be estimated that treating 1,000 middle-aged men with hypercholesterolemia and no evidence of a previous myocardial infarction with pravastatin for five years will result in . . . seven fewer deaths from cardiovascular causes, and two fewer deaths from other causes than would be expected in the absence of treatment."

And one more thing: it's important to remember that the WOSCOPS trial was heavily populated with high-risk patients. Even then the statins didn't help all that much, and no one knows how many of them experienced statin-related adverse effects that weren't detected or reported.

Most subsequent studies of statins haven't demonstrated better results than the 1996 WOSCOPS trial. Some studies, in fact, have found statins to be all but useless in terms of primary prevention — which, as noted earlier, is why 75 percent of the prescriptions for statins are written in the first place.

Statins have a checkered history. The first statin to be marketed as a cholesterol-lowering agent was triparanol (MER-29), which the Food and Drug Administration approved in 1959. It was withdrawn from the market three years later. As it turned out, the drug's manufacturer had falsified the data it had submitted to the FDA to hide the fact that its product caused cataracts in rats and dogs in preclinical trials. Humans who later took triparanol developed the same unusual form of cataracts and went blind. The drug company and three of its executives later pleaded no contest to supplying the FDA with "false, fictitious, and fraudulent" data.

The scandal undoubtedly dampened the interest of pharmaceutical companies in the commercial potential of statin drugs. But in 1976, Japanese researchers isolated another cholesterol-inhibiting compound, compactin, and by 1979, Merck scientists had, in turn, isolated lovastatin from it. The FDA approved lovastatin in 1987.

Now, all these years later, we are really just beginning to learn more about statins and their adverse effects, especially on older people.

In 2010, for example, the highly respected Cochrane Collaboration systematically reviewed twenty-two randomized, controlled trials of statin drugs. And when its researchers adjusted for various forms of bias — such as the unnoted inclusion of secondary prevention patients in trials — the purported mortality benefits of statins began to disappear.

The Cochrane review's conclusions were nothing short of startling. "The claimed mortality benefit of statins for primary prevention is more likely a measure of bias than a real effect," the authors wrote. Their bottom line? "Statins do not have a proven net health benefit in primary prevention populations."

Thus I feel I'm on solid footing in viewing statins as drugs of last resort, all the more so because nondrug approaches can be effective in controlling a patient's lipid levels without all the baggage that statins put on board.

For starters, it's important to identify and then eliminate, if at all possible, other risk factors for cardiovascular disease, such as smoking and excess weight.

I advise patients to avoid foods that are high in saturated fat — that alone can drop your LDL level by 5 percent or so — and to add lots of fiber-rich foods to their diets. And there's some evidence that lycopene, the powerful antioxidant that gives ripe tomatoes their bright red color, may be especially helpful. A team of Australian researchers reported in 2011 that eating as little as two ounces of tomato paste a day could be an effective alternative to statins: "Our meta-analysis suggests," they wrote, "that lycopene taken in doses of at least 25 milligrams daily is effective in reducing LDL cholesterol by about 10 percent, which is comparable to the effect of low doses of statins in patients with slightly elevated cholesterol levels."

Exercise is especially important, as it's probably the best way to boost HDL levels. Inactive people who take up some form of regular physical activity can expect to see their HDL levels increase by as much as 20 percent. Moderate alcohol consumption (one or two drinks a day) can help a little bit too.

Above all, though, I find that a combination of vitamin B_{12}, folic acid, vitamin B_6, and omega-3 fish oil is an effective approach to lipid control in older patients. Scientific evidence suggests that fish oil lowers high triglycerides and, in recommended amounts, seems to help prevent heart disease and stroke. There's also evidence that vitamin B_{12} in combination with fish oil may be more effective than fish oil alone in reducing triglycerides and total blood cholesterol.

Older people need to be given vitamin B_{12} by injection — or, as a second choice, sublingually (under the tongue) — in order to receive any benefits from it. At around age forty-five, our stomachs no longer produce an enzyme known as intrinsic factor (IF), which is essential for absorbing vitamin B^{12}. I typically recommend 1,000 micrograms of vitamin B_{12} by injection into the muscle each week for four weeks, then going to monthly, along with a daily regimen of folic acid (1 milligram), vitamin B_6 (200 milligrams), and fish oil (3,000 milligrams). Older patients should maintain a blood B_{12} level of around 1,000, which, recent studies show, improves both muscle tone and cognition.

If you're sixty or older, my recommendation is that you stay away from statins at all costs — the greatest cost, of course, being your good health.

DOWN AND OUT:
DRUG-INDUCED FALLS

A fall can kill you, especially if you're older.

Each year, one in three Americans aged sixty-five or older falls. In this age group, falls are the number one cause of injuries, deaths from injury, and hospital admissions for trauma.

Of all older Americans who fall each year, 20 percent to 30 percent suffer moderate to severe injuries that make it hard for them to get around or live independently and increase their risk of dying early. Some studies show that the life expectancy of older patients with repeated falls is only about eighteen months.

Falls present an enormous public health problem. In 2009, emergency departments across the nation treated 2.2 million nonfatal fall injuries among older adults, according to the Centers for Disease Control and Prevention, and more than 582,000 of these patients had to be hospitalized.

The older you are, the higher the risk. And if you're no longer living at home, the risk is higher yet. Up to half of all people in long-term care facilities fall each year, and 40 percent of them fall repeatedly.

Nursing homes and other long-term care facilities are required to report all falls. But when people living at home fall, the incident becomes part of the statistics only if they end up in the emergency room or otherwise receive medical attention for their injuries. My experience in both institutional and outpatient settings tells me that the incidence of falls is much greater when people are on their own, outside of the controlled environment of a long-term care facility.

Falls can result in lacerations and skin tears, wrist and arm fractures, hip fractures, traumatic brain injuries (such as bleeding around the brain), and injuries to other internal organs. If you sustain a hip fracture from a fall, danger looms: one in five hip-fracture patients dies within a year of their injuries.

What's so tragic about this epidemic is that it is largely preventable. I know this from more than forty years of clinical experience, and I know that the real cause of most falls goes undetected or unrecorded.

When I see patients who have experienced

one or more falls, I immediately know to look at the list of medications that they're taking, both on doctor's orders and on their own. As sure as the sun sets in the west, I know that somewhere in that list I'm likely to find the cause. More than 95 percent of the time I do.

A bewildering array of medications — prescription and nonprescription — can cause falls, either on their own or in concert with other drugs and events.

Suppose for a moment that you're in the grocery store and happen to think about the occasional episodes of insomnia you've been having lately. As you look at the scores of available sleep aids, you see Extra Strength Tylenol PM (acetaminophen and diphenhydramine) — the one with a crescent moon and stars on the package, right next to the words *Non-habit forming.* Maybe this, you think, will help you get to sleep tonight. Is it safe? Well, it has to be, you say to yourself, or they wouldn't sell it without a prescription. So you drop it into your shopping cart and buy it along with your groceries.

If you're sixty or older, you may have just bought your ticket to a fall or perhaps even a broken bone.

Most people know the diphenhydramine that's in Tylenol PM — and Advil PM and Excedrin PM and nearly all the other PM products — by the brand name Benadryl. A first-generation antihistamine, diphenhydramine has powerful sedative properties and thus is an ingredient in many nonprescription sleep aids. (It is also available in stand-alone form under such brand names as Sleep-ettes, Sleep-eze, Sleepinal, Sominex, Somnicaps, and Unisom.) Sometimes I even see doctors prescribe 50 milligrams of diphenhydramine at bedtime for eighty-year-olds.

The falls often occur when older people take a diphenhydramine-containing product to go to sleep and then get up at night to go to the bathroom. The drug's strong sedative powers have lowered their blood pressure; as they stand, they experience some or all of the classic effects of central nervous system depression: blurred vision, impaired thinking, unsteadiness, slowed reflexes, and perhaps the loss of consciousness. At some point before they reach the bathroom, they fall.

Allergy medicines carry the same risk. Suppose, for a moment, that your seventy-one-year-old father is taking tamsulosin (Flomax), an alpha-blocker, for benign prostatic hyperplasia (BPH). It's the height of hay fever season, and he sees a commercial on television that portrays chlorpheniramine (Chlor-Trimeton) as a gentle way to stop his sneezing and congestion. He can buy it without a prescription, and his thought is to use it to relieve his symptoms until the pollen count goes down.

What he doesn't know is that, at his age, he lacks the kidney function needed to clear the tamsulosin from his body in a timely manner. Adding chlorpheniramine on top of an alpha-blocker can make things much worse — as his kidneys struggle unsuccessfully to clear an even higher drug load — and cause serious problems with balance. The result, as it plays out in your father's case, is orthostatic hypotension, although he doesn't realize that the dizziness he experiences when he stands up is a side effect of the drugs he's taking.

A few days later, your father needs to change a lightbulb in the hallway and steps up on a chair to reach the fixture on the ceiling. He basically passes out and falls off the chair, but because he lives alone, no one is around to help or call an ambulance. A day later, he's in the hospital, and it will be many months before he's back where he was before the accident. No one realizes that the antihistamine had anything to do with his fall.

Then there's the retired salesman who has type 2 diabetes and takes chlorpropamide (Diabinese) every morning to control his blood sugar. Chlorpropamide, a member of the sulfonylurea class of antidiabetic drugs, has been on the market for more than fifty years. His doctor has been prescribing the medication for so long that he's not even aware of a warning added to the package insert in 2002 concerning its use in older patients: "The safety and effectiveness of Diabinese in patients aged sixty-five and over has not been properly evaluated in clinical studies. Chlorpropamide remains on a list of drugs that are inappropriate for use in older adults because it can cause prolonged low blood sugar [hypoglycemia]."

One morning, after eating a light breakfast and taking his morning medications, the man finishes reading the newspaper and then hops into the shower to get ready for a round of golf. He doesn't know it, but his blood sugar has dropped precipitously, and the hypoglycemia causes him to lose consciousness. He falls in the shower, breaks his arm, and bruises some ribs. His wife calls 911, and soon he is rushed to the hospital in an ambulance. Everyone assumes that he slipped in the shower, and the Diabinese is never implicated in his accident.

The more medications you take, the greater your risk of a fall. And with so many older people taking five or more medications, it's a wonder that there aren't more falls. As William Dalziel, MD, a prominent Canadian geriatrician, puts it, "You'd fall down, too, if you were on so many drugs."

In my practice, one of my top priorities is always looking for ways to prevent drug-induced falls. For most older people, a fall is a life-changing experience. Some wrongly take it as a sign that they are getting too old to exercise or to participate in other normal activities. Some worry that their families or other loved ones will rush to the conclusion that they can no longer live on their own and that they need to be in a nursing home or similar setting. Some develop such an extreme fear of falling that they come to live, with each passing month, in greater isolation. And some simply quit taking the medicine that they feel might have caused or contributed to the fall, which may put their health in even greater jeopardy.

Over the years, I've seen it all. And often all it takes is one drug-triggered fall to set off a long chain of other events — pretty much like a row of dominos tipping over in sequence.

When I see an older person taking a medication that's known to increase the risk of falls, I know to do one of three things: (1) discontinue the drug unless its benefit outweighs the risk; (2) lower the dosage to the maximum extent possible without losing the therapeutic effect; or (3) find another medication or therapy that helps the patient without exposing him or her to the risk. In my experience, nondrug therapies are an especially attractive alternative to antidepressants, many of which don't do much better than placebo in clinical trials and elevate the patient's risk of a fall by as much as 70 percent.

A federal task force recently reviewed the results of fifty-four clinical trials to identify the most effective ways to reduce the risk of falling in people sixty-five and older. Its report, published in the *Annals of Internal Medicine* in 2010, found that vitamin D supplementation reduces the risk of falls by 17 percent (by helping to build stronger muscles) and that exercise or physical therapy reduces the risk of falls by 13 percent.

I recommend that older people take at

least 700 to 1,000 IU (international units) of supplemental vitamin D daily. It's important to let your physician or pharmacist know that you're doing this, and to have the vitamin D concentration in your blood measured at least once a year, as vitamin D can build up and cause problems in some people.

If you or someone you love should suffer a fall, no matter how trivial it might seem at the time, the early intervention of a consultant pharmacist can make all the difference in ensuring that it doesn't happen again. And the difference may be one of life or death.

The medications associated most directly with falls are those that act as central nervous system (CNS) depressants, such as benzodiazepines (used widely to treat anxiety and sleep disorders), sedatives, and tranquilizers. Older people are most vulnerable to their CNS-related effects because various age-related physiologic changes — decreased muscle mass and diminished kidney and liver functions, for example — directly affect how their bodies absorb, distribute, metabolize, and eliminate these drugs.

The classes of medications most often responsible for falls that lead to hip fractures are antipsychotics (52 percent), sleeping pills and minor tranquilizers (30 percent), and antidepressants (17 percent). Drugs in all of these classes are often prescribed unnecessarily, especially in older adults. Each year, according to one study, 32,000 older adults sustain hip fractures that are attributable to drug-induced falls, resulting in more than 1,500 deaths.

Many, many other classes of drugs can lead to falls by causing impaired balance and reaction time, light-headedness, dizziness, drowsiness, hypotension, sedation, and other such effects.

Here's a checklist of medications that can cause you to fall (and why):

Analgesics (especially opioids). These drugs are CNS depressants that can reduce your alertness or leave you feeling light-headed, dizzy, and faint.

Examples (including combinations with acetaminophen): fentanyl (Duragesic), hydrocodone (Norco, Vicodin), hydromorphone (Dilaudid, Exalgo), morphine (Astramorph, Avinza), oxycodone (OxyContin, Percocet).

Antiarrhythmics. These drugs, which are used to treat abnormal heart rhythms, can impair the flow of blood to the brain, causing dizziness, light-headedness, and fainting.

Examples: amiodarone (Cordarone), flecainide (Tambocor), procainamide (Procanbid), sotalol (Betapace).

Antibiotics and other anti-infective agents. Some of these medications can disturb your balance by damaging the inner ear.

Examples: ciprofloxacin (Ciloxan, Cipro), enoxacin (Penetrex), gemifloxacin (Factive), levofloxacin (Levaquin), lomefloxacin (Maxaquin), mebendazole (Vermox), moxifloxacin (Avelox), norfloxacin (Chibroxin, Noroxin), ofloxacin (Floxin, Ocuflox), sparfloxacin (Zagam).

Anticonvulsants. These drugs can impair your balance, coordination, and gait, and can cause confusion and drowsiness.

In the event that an anticonvulsant is absolutely necessary, then the lowest dose possible needs to be established with close monitoring of the individual's tolerance to the drug. Often I see patients on such excessive doses of anticonvulsants that their drug-induced cognitive impairment is mistaken for Alzheimer's disease and thus isn't recognized as a drug effect. In such cases falls are almost a certainty.

Examples: carbamazepine (Tegretol), clonazepam (Klonopin), lamotrigine (Lamictal), phenytoin (Dilantin), valproate (Epilim).

Antidepressants. Many studies have linked antidepressants — especially tricyclic antidepressants and selective serotonin re-uptake inhibitors (SSRIs) — to falls, as they can cause daytime drowsiness, impaired sleep, insomnia, nocturia (the need to get up in the night to urinate), impaired reflexes and reaction times, orthostatic hypotension, and movement disorders, among other conditions. All can be contributing factors in falls.

Another problem with antidepressants is that many of them require the liver isozyme CYP2D6 to metabolize, and 50 percent to 60 percent of older people do not make that isozyme anymore. The drug then ends up in the liver without the proper pathway to break down, frequently causing problems with other drugs being taken at the same time, and further increasing the risk for syncope (fainting) and serious falls.

Examples: amitriptyline (Elavil), amitriptyline-chlordiazepoxide (Limbitrol), amitriptyline-perphenazine (Triavil), amoxapine (Asendin), bupropion (Wellbutrin), citalopram (Celexa), desipramine (Norpramin), doxepin (Sinequan), escitalopram (Lexapro), fluoxetine (Prozac, Sarafem), fluvoxamine (Luvox), imipramine (Tofranil), maprotiline (Ludiomil), nortriptyline (Aventyl, Pamelor), paroxetine (Paxil), sertraline (Zoloft), trazodone (Desyrel).

Antihistamines. Cold, cough, allergy, and asthma medications that contain antihistamines can cause sedation and psychomotor impairment. In high enough doses, some can cause hypotension.

While you won't find the word *falls* on the package insert for Benadryl, for example, you will see this sentence: "Antihistamines are more likely to cause dizziness, sedation, and hypotension in elderly patients." Those are the ingredients of a fall.

Although hydroxyzine (Atarax, Vistaril) is prescribed a lot to younger people as an antianxiety drug, in the older patient it almost always has the opposite effect, along with all the serious anticholinergic side effects that cause falls (blurred vision, confusion, syncope, and so on).

Examples: azatadine (Optimine), brompheniramine (Dimetane), chlorpheniramine (Alermine, Chlor-Trimeton), clemastine (Tavist, Tavist-1), cyproheptadine (Periactin), dextromethorphan (Delsym), diphenhydramine (Benadryl, Sominex), hydroxyzine (Atarax, Vistaril), triprolidine (Myidil).

Antihypertensives. As medications prescribed to lower your blood pressure, antihypertensives bring with them the heightened risk of orthostatic hypotension: a sudden drop in blood pressure triggered by a change in body position. The drop in blood pressure causes a shortage of oxygen to the brain, leading to light-headedness, dizziness, and sometimes blackouts.

Orthostatic hypotension — also called postural hypotension — is extremely common in older people and can also lead to altered perceptions, problems with coordination and movement mobility, and poor balance. All of these, of course, are key ingredients for falls. And often all of these adverse effects are most pronounced in the first few weeks of taking the drugs — just when the patient may be least prepared for them.

Examples: atenolol (Noten, Tenormin), carvedilol (Coreg), enalapril (Vasotec), felo-

dipine (Felodur, Plendil/Felodur), meto-
prolol (Betaloc, Lopressor), nifedipine
(Adalat Oros), ramipril (Tritace), sotalol
(Betapace), verapamil (Anpec, Isoptin).

Antiparkinsonian drugs. These drugs can
impair a patient's balance, coordination,
and gait as well as cause light-headedness,
dizziness, confusion, and hallucinations.

The use of dopamine receptor agonists in
older patients puts them on an almost
certain path to falls. In my practice, I typically see these drugs prescribed to treat restless leg syndrome (RLS), a condition that
in most cases is caused by the use of statins
or other drugs. With dopamine receptor
agonists, a warning sign is sudden, excessive daytime sleepiness.

Monoamine oxidase type B (MAO-B)
inhibitors, which are also used to treat the
symptoms of Parkinson's disease, can pose
even larger problems in terms of falls. These
drugs are not recommended for older patients because they can cause severe orthostatic hypotension, psychotic disorders, tardive dyskinesia (an irreversible neurological
disorder characterized by involuntary and
repetitive movements such as grimacing and
tongue thrusting), and excessive tremors.

Because falls are such a frequent complication of Parkinson's disease, the risk-benefit equation for some of the antiparkinsonian drugs can be tricky to evaluate. Studies have linked two classic Parkinson's symptoms — rigidity and bradykinesia (a slowness in the execution of movement) — to falls, so the drugs may help with those symptoms at the same time that their side effects heighten risks in other areas.

Above all, it's important to remember that if you or a loved one has any of the symptoms of parkinsonism, there's a good chance that they're really being caused by drugs. Studies suggest, in fact, that as much as half of all parkinsonism in older adults is drug induced. Here are several examples:

Dopamine receptor agonists: bromocriptine (Parlodel), pramipexole (Mirapex), ropinirole (Requip)
L-dopa: levodopa (Larodopa), carbidopa-levodopa (Sinemet)
MAO-B inhibitors: selegiline (Eldepryl)

Antipsychotics. All of the antipsychotic drugs can cause tardive dyskinesia and other movement disorders, sedation, unsteadiness in walking and other forms of psychomotor retardation, cognitive impairment, postural hypotension, orthostatic hypotension, blurred vision, fainting, and, with long-term usage, parkinsonism.

Antipsychotic drugs increase the risk of falls, especially in older people, and especially when used with other drugs, which older people are far more likely to do than younger people.

If you're an older person who's taking an antipsychotic drug, the question isn't so much whether you're going to fall, but when and how often. Whenever I don't see any falls noted in the charts of patients who've been taking these medications, in fact, I know to be skeptical. It's a virtual certainty, in my experience, that there were falls that didn't make it into their medical histories for one reason or another.

Many people believe that antipsychotic drugs aren't used as widely in nursing homes as they used to be, but, in fact, the opposite is true. The percentage of elderly patients in nursing homes who are given antipsychotic drugs has increased dramatically from 16.4 percent in 1996 to 25.9 percent in 2006.

Guidelines published in 2010 by the American Geriatrics Society, the British Geriatrics Society, and the American Academy of Orthopaedic Surgeons Panel on Falls Prevention recommend that patients who have fallen may benefit from the discontinuation of antipsychotics and other psychotropic medications.

There are big questions as to the true value of these drugs in the treatment of older patients with dementia of any type. I generally find that these medications can be reduced drastically or discontinued. The key is to create an environment that is familiar and comforting to the patient, and, if needed, using one of the newer antianxiety-antidepressant combination drugs. In my experience, these changes remove most if not all of the serious side effects of the antipsychotic drugs — including falls.

Examples: amitriptyline-perphenazine (Triavil), aripiprazole (Abilify), chlorpromazine (Thorazine), clozapine (Clozaril), fluphenazine (Prolixin), haloperidol (Haldol), olanzapine (Zyprexa), prochlorperazine (Compazine), risperidone (Risperdal), thioridazine (Mellaril), thiothixene (Navane), trifluoperazine (Stelazine), ziprasidone (Geodon).

Beta-blockers. Beta-blockers typically aren't the best choice for treating cardiovascular problems in older adults. That's because nearly half of all people sixty and older don't produce the CYP2D6 liver enzyme needed to properly metabolize the drug. As the beta-blocker builds up in a patient's system, all the adverse effects commonly associated with its use are exacerbated, including insomnia, dizziness, and vertigo — all of which are contributing factors in falls.

Examples: acebutolol (Sectral), atenolol (Tenormin), betaxolol (Kerlone), bisoprolol (Zebeta), carvedilol (Coreg), metoprolol (Lopressor, Toprol), nadolol (Corgard), penbutolol (Levatol), pindolol (Visken), propranolol (Inderal), timolol (Blocadren).

Corticosteroids. Corticosteroids used in high doses or for long periods of time and then stopped abruptly can cause many serious central nervous system problems, leading to falls.

Examples: dexamethasone (Decadron, Hexadrol, Mymethasone), hydrocortisone (Cortef, Hydrocortone), methylprednisolone (Medrol), prednisolone (Prelone), prednisone (Deltasone).

Diuretics. Diuretics can cause nocturia as well as postural hypotension and orthostatic hypotension.

A study released at a 2011 meeting of the American Geriatrics Society showed that nursing home residents who are started on a diuretic or are put on a higher dose of a diuretic "have an acute surge in their fall risk."

Examples: amiloride-hydrochlorothiazide (Moduretic), amiloride (Midamor), furosemide (Lasix, Uremide), indapamide (Dapa-tabs, Natrilix), spironolactone (Aldactone).

Muscle relaxants. It may surprise you to learn that these drugs do not directly relax muscles; they are central nervous system (CNS) depressants that act as sedatives. They can trigger falls by impairing a patient's balance, coordination, and gait — the typical anticholinergic effects of all CNS depressants — and causing drowsiness, sedation, and altered perception.

"The decision to prescribe muscle relaxants for elderly people should take into account the risk of severe fracture associated with these drugs," concluded a study published in the journal *BMC Geriatrics* in 2008.

All these drugs are contraindicated in older patients because their side effects can be so serious. Cyclobenzaprine (Flexeril), for example, can cause severe hallucinations in older patients, and it has the highest morbidity rate of any drug in the older-patient population.

Examples: baclofen (Gablofen, Kemstro, Lioresal), carisoprodol (Soma), chlorzoxazone (Parafon, Relax), cyclobenzaprine (Flexeril), diazepam (Valium), methocarbamol (Robaxin), orphenadrine (Norflex).

Nitrates. These drugs, which are used to treat acute angina (severe chest pain or discomfort), can cause dizziness, light-headedness, and fainting. Because older people have reduced function of baroreceptors — sensors in the body that regulate blood pressure — the use of nitrates can cause severe orthostatic hypotension.

Examples: isosorbide dinitrate (Dilatrate, Sorbitrate), isosorbide-5-mononitrate (Ismo, Monoket), nitroglycerin (Minitran, Nitro-Bid, Nitro-Dur, Nitrostat).

Nonsteroidal anti-inflammatory drugs (NSAIDs). NSAIDs increase the risk of falls through a variety of adverse central nervous system (CNS) effects, including confusion, dizziness, light-headedness, drowsiness, and vision impairment.

The use of NSAIDs has long been associated with an increased risk of falls. A review of the published studies that appeared in the journal *Drug Safety* in 2009 concluded that, despite some imperfections and ambiguities, "all studies showed an increased risk of falling due to NSAID use."

Examples: etodolac (Lodine), ibuprofen (Motrin, Advil, Medipren), flurbiprofen (Ansaid, Ocufen), ketoprofen (Orudis), naproxen (Anaprox, Naprosyn, Aleve), indomethacin (Indocin), ketorolac (Toradol).

Ophthalmic beta-blockers. Most people think of eye drops as being harmless, but this class of drugs — typically prescribed to treat the symptoms of glaucoma — is anything but. Even a low dose of an ophthalmic beta-blocker can cause severe systemic adverse effects.

I've seen patients, for example, who've had asthma attacks from one drop of these drugs being placed in an eye. Other problems associated with beta-blockers — dizziness and vertigo, for example — can lead to falls. Although the medication does lower intraocular pressure (the fluid pressure inside the eye), it often comes with unwanted side effects: from the worsening of respiratory problems, to depression, hallucinations, and cognitive changes. There are so many other medications to lower the intraocular pressure associated with glaucoma effectively and safely that these drugs, in my judgment, should never even be considered, especially in older people.

An article published in the *British Medical Journal* in 2006 concluded, "Eye drops with beta-blocking action can have a strong and prolonged systemic effect, especially in older age groups. Beta-blocker eye drops should be prescribed with caution in older patients and in patients with preexisting cardiovascular morbidity."

Examples: carteolol (Cartrol), levobunolol (Betagan), metipranolol (Optipranolol), timolol (Timoptic).

Sulfonylurea drugs. This class of drugs, the first type of oral medication used to treat type 2 diabetes, has been around since the mid-1950s. All of the sulfonylureas, especially the long-acting ones, can increase the risk of falls by inducing hypoglycemia, or low blood sugar.

Low blood sugar, in fact, is the most common side effect of the sulfonylurea drugs. Package inserts for the drugs note that all of them "are capable of producing severe hypoglycemia, which may result in coma, and may require hospitalization." And older people who use these medications are at the greatest risk because of their impaired renal function.

There are so many other drugs available to treat type 2 diabetes that the use of the sulfonylureas in older patients, in my judgment, is always inadvisable.

A study published in 2011 found that diabetic patients treated for five to eight years with diet plus the sulfonylurea drug tolbutamide (Orinase) were two and a half times more likely to suffer a fatal cardiovascular event than patients treated with diet alone. The government warning noted that while tolbutamide was the only sulfonylurea drug included in the study, "it is prudent from a safety standpoint to consider that this warning may also apply to other oral hypoglycemic drugs in this class, in view of their close similarities in mode of action and chemical structure."

Tranquilizers and sleeping pills. These drugs, as sedatives, are powerful central nervous system (CNS) depressants. They can trigger falls by impairing a patient's balance, coordination, and gait and by causing drowsiness and altered perception. Common sense suggests that any drug that will tranquilize you or put you to sleep can also put you at risk of a fall.

Most of these drugs are in the benzodiazepine family. Some have long half-lives and some have shorter half-lives, but all are long acting in older patients because they lack the hepatic isozymes to metabolize the drugs. For this reason, you have residual amounts of the drug lingering and then being compounded by additional doses. The result is syncope and serious falls.

The fall-related dangers of benzodiazepines have been known for many years. A 1997 study, for example, reported, "For men and women 60 years and older, a first benzodiazepine prescription is associated with an increased risk of hospitalization for a fall, and the risk of hospitalization for an injurious fall is highest in the first two weeks of drug use."

Examples: chloral hydrate (Noctec), chlordiazepoxide (Librium), clorazepate (Tranxene), diazepam (Valium), etchlorvynol (Placidyl), flurazepam (Dalmane), glutethimide (Doriden), hydroxyzine (Atarax, Vistaril), lorazepam (Ativan), meprobamate (Miltown, Equanil), methyprylon (Noludar), oxazepam (Serax), prazepam (Centrax), temazepam (Restoril), triazolam (Halcion), zaleplon (Sonata, Starnoc), zolpidem (Ambien).

THE BONE-SCARE DRUGS: WHAT YOU SHOULD KNOW ABOUT BISPHOSPHONATES

Let's start with a fundamental truth: as you grow older, your bones grow weaker.

You may not have realized it, but the bones in your body are actually alive. Indeed, they are complex organs that are changing constantly. Every day, old bone cells die and new ones are created to take their place. When we're young, our bodies create lots and lots of new bone cells to help us grow. When we reach a certain age — for most of us, it's somewhere in our mid-thirties — our bodies produce just enough new bone cells to replace the bone cells we're losing. Unfortunately, this stage of relative equilibrium isn't destined to last very long. As we age further, and as our bodies undergo other changes, the bone-renewal process slows down to the point where our bodies can't create new bone cells fast enough to make up for the lost bone cells.

The cells that form new bone are called osteoblasts, while the cells that break down and clear out the old cells are called osteoclasts. This little bit of chemistry is worth knowing, and we'll be coming back to it shortly. For now, though, the important thing to remember is that what nature gives us when we're young — bones that are growing stronger by the day — it begins to start taking away, in microscopic increments, as we age. It's a fact of life, and of growing older, that we can't change.

Sadly, however, as far as I am concerned, millions of older people (mostly older women) have been duped into thinking that one or another of the prescription drugs known as bisphosphonates — marketed under such brand names as risedronate (Actone), ibandronate (Boniva), aldrenate (Fosamax), and zoledronic acid (Reclast) — are a miracle cure for bone loss. Since their introduction in 1995, in fact, bisphosphonates have become big moneymakers for pharmaceutical companies, and today they rank among the top-selling drugs in the United States.

Turn on the television or leaf through a magazine, and chances are you'll see a commercial or advertisement warning you about bone loss. The ads all ask basically the same question (What can you do about bone loss?) and suggest the same answer (take a prescription drug).

Most of us can easily picture actress Sally Field doing exactly that in her role as spokeswoman for Boniva, which is marketed in the United States by the Roche Group's Genentech subsidiary. "Boniva did more than stop my bone loss," she says in a typical ad. "It worked with my body to reverse it!" In interviews, Field has gone so far as to call the drug "a miracle."

I think of Boniva as anything but a miracle, however, and for some women — those who experience spontaneous fractures of their hip bone or learn that their jawbones are slowly and irreversibly dissolving — the bisphosphonates may be more on the order of nightmare drugs.

There's no question that osteoporosis — a decrease in bone density — is relatively common among older adults. Because the bone disorder is estimated to cause more than 1.5 million fractures a year, including more than 300,000 hip fractures, it needs to be taken seriously. But are bisphosphonate drugs like Boniva the right approach to treating the disease? I don't think so.

In all too many cases (at least the ones I

see), a woman goes to see her doctor and leaves with a prescription for a bisphosphonate simply because the bone scan that her doctor ordered shows that her "T-score" — the number of standard deviations below the average for a young adult at peak bone density — is minus 1 or lower. A lot of doctors, in fact, are sold on the idea of prescribing bisphosphonate drugs prophylactically — namely, to prevent osteoporosis.

The scan-and-prescribe approach, in my judgment, is cookbook medicine at its worst. Here's why.

With my patients, the first thing I always want to know is whether there's something other than age that can be causing the bone loss. Often there is. Many years ago, for example, my mother was prescribed massive injections of corticosteroid drugs for her osteoarthritis. Some of us will remember that cortisone was trumpeted as "a miracle drug." As it turned out, it wasn't, and millions of American women, including my mother, experienced severe bone loss from taking corticosteroids. In her case, the cortisone basically caused her bones to completely dissolve over time.

All forms of steroid medications can bring about bone loss, especially if you take them at high doses or for a long time. Because of their anti-inflammatory and antiallergic effects, steroids are used to treat rheumatoid arthritis, lupus, respiratory disease, asthma, allergies, and many other conditions. So one of the first things I want to know is whether my patients are taking some form of steroid; if they are, I want them to stop. But, as with many medications, there's a problem. Discontinuing steroids abruptly in patients who have been on them for a long time typically causes severe withdrawal symptoms and can even be fatal, owing to the fact that the normal production of steroids by the body has been turned off. As a result, the patient typically needs to be tapered slowly off the steroid medication.

Lots of other drugs will cause bone loss. Short-acting loop diuretics, for example, which are typically prescribed to treat hypertension (high blood pressure) and edema (fluid retention), have been associated with increased rates of hip-bone loss, and they're among the medications prescribed most commonly to older adults.

Proton pump inhibitors — drugs such as esomeprazole (Nexium), lansoprazole (Prevacid), omeprazole (Prilosec), and pantoprazole (Protonix), which are used typically to treat the symptoms of gastroesophageal reflux disease (GERD) — bring the absorption of calcium in a patient's body to a sudden stop. This can lead to bone breaks in the hip and spine after as little as one year of therapy. A study published in the *Journal of the American Medical Association* in 2006 found that patients fifty years of age and older who took these drugs for more than a year had a 44 percent increased risk of breaking a hip. And long-term PPI therapy, the study revealed, increased the risk of hip fracture by as much as 245 percent.

Similarly, some diseases and other health problems can cause bone loss, so it's important that they're factored into the patient's equation.

The next thing I want to know is whether patients really understand the risks of taking bisphosphonate drugs. Nearly always, I find that they are totally unaware of the risks or believe the risks to be remote, based on the fact that their doctors didn't mention any as they wrote the prescriptions.

When I talk to patients about the bisphosphonate drugs — and usually it's to talk them out of taking them — these are the risks I'm careful to cover:

Pain in your muscles, joints, and bones. When I meet with someone who's been taking a bisphosphonate drug, I always ask if she has any pains that she didn't have before. In response to my question, I often hear stories of pain so severe that the person has stopped running, working out, or some other activity with health benefits. "Do you think it has something to do with the drug?" I'm typically asked. My standard reply: "It's probably the drug that's causing the pain."

I don't know why people are so shocked to hear this, but they are. Often they don't want to believe that a drug their physician tells them they need could actually be harming them. As we've seen, however, doctors are often unaware of common adverse effects linked to the drugs they're prescribing.

You don't have to take my word for this. When the Food and Drug Administration issued a warning that bisphosphonate drugs may lead to severe, chronic, and even permanent pain in muscles, joints, and bones, it specifically emphasized that many doctors did not appear to be aware that the drugs could cause such pain in their patients. The FDA's warning pointed out that patients could develop severe pain "within days" after starting on a bisphosphonate drug and that the pain could be intense enough to interfere with such routine day-to-day activities as climbing stairs. (And you tell me: Are you more likely to fall on the stairs and break a bone because you're losing a tiny bit of bone density year by year or because you're in a lot of pain as you struggle to navigate your way up and down?)

In my experience, when these patients go back to their doctors to ask about the pain, they're told that the pain is from their osteoporosis or "pre-osteoporosis," and not from the drug they've been prescribed. Some of these patients then begin self-medicating by taking over-the-counter preparations for the pain, which is about the worst thing they can possibly do.

An article in the *Archives of Internal Medicine* on the experiences of patients taking Fosamax found that doctors often responded to those experiencing severe pain by putting them through numerous — and, it turned out, generally needless — diagnostic tests. A majority of the patients experienced gradual and sometimes even immediate relief from their pain after the drug was discontinued.

Gastrointestinal problems. The most common adverse effects of bisphosphonates are gastrointestinal. They range from heartburn, acid reflux, and other relatively mild GI events to inflammation (esophagitis), ulcerations, and even cancer of the esophagus.

To me, the heightened cancer risk associated with bisphosphonates far outweighs whatever possible benefits might be claimed for them. A study published in the *British Medical Journal* in September 2010 showed that patients who took bisphosphonates for five years or filled at least ten prescriptions for the drugs were twice as likely to be diagnosed with esophageal cancer as those who didn't.

Although a study published in the *Journal of the American Medical Association* a month earlier concluded that there was no link between bisphosphonates and esophageal cancer, I'd judge the British study as far more authoritative because it tracked patients for nearly twice as long (almost eight years).

Additionally, as I see very old patients come into the nursing home on a bisphosphonate drug, eight out of ten have some degree of erosive esophagitis, which, if I can't get the doctor to stop the drug, often leads to fatal outcomes.

Spontaneous bone fractures. You may have read or heard the stories of women who, after taking bisphosphonates for a number of years, fractured their hip bone while simply walking or standing. While these low-trauma and nontraumatic fractures are uncommon, it tells us that there's something about how the drugs work that we still don't understand. It also suggests that bisphosphonate-triggered bone resorption may not actually give women stronger bones over time and, in fact, may make their bones more brittle.

TIME BOMB DRUGS?

I'm not sold on the theory that bisphosphonate drugs make bone stronger. We don't know yet whether denser bone — as measured by a bone scan — is actually stronger bone. But we do know that bisphosphonate drugs, while doing the "good" that they are supposed to do, also stop the body's natural ability to repair bone. Is it possible that using these drugs for many years causes the bones to be weakened rather than strengthened? No one knows. And that's something really worth thinking about before you start taking a bisphosphonate drug.

I do know, as a pharmacotherapist, that rebound effects are common with many prescription (and nonprescription) drugs. A rebound effect (or "rebound phenomenon") is what happens when the body tries to

309

bring itself back into balance after a drug alters or stops one of its internal processes: simply put, it pulls in the opposite direction of the drug, and sometimes overcompensates violently before seeking equilibrium.

Bone strength encompasses bone density and bone quality, but doctors tend to diagnose osteoporosis solely on bone density, as measured by a DXA (which stands for dual X-ray absorptiometry) scan. The machine does this by passing a dual energy X-ray beam through the patient's body. But low bone density, as measured by DXA scans, is an imperfect predictor of fracture risk — so imperfect, in fact, that it identifies fewer than half the people who will eventually suffer an osteoporotic fracture. That's why the scan-and-prescribe approach, in my judgment, is so deeply flawed.

Jawbone deterioration. Bisphosphonate drugs, in rare cases, can cause osteonecrosis of the jaw, or "jaw death." Although the literature suggests that this frightening adverse event is rare, as time goes on with the experience of this drug, it becomes more common day by day. With osteonecrosis, a bone is no longer alive and cannot regenerate because of a lack of blood supply. In May 2010 a New York jury awarded $8 million in damages to a seventy-two-year-old Florida woman who said that she'd developed osteonecrosis of the jaw from taking Fosamax. Many more cases are lined up behind hers.

The first large population-based study to look at the relationship between bisphosphonates and osteonecrosis of the jaw was published in 2009 — nearly fifteen years after Fosamax was approved for the market. It found that 4 percent of the patients taking Fosamax were being treated for active osteonecrosis of the jaw, as opposed to zero percent of people not taking it. Even short-term use of the drug, according to the study, increased the risk.

Another big problem I see is the increasing use of bisphosphonate infusions — basically, the intravenous administration of the drug — to provide a year's worth of therapy with one procedure, at which point another infusion will be administered. What if three months after you receive your first infusion you discover osteonecrosis in your jaw, need an invasive dental procedure, or are diagnosed with erosive esophagitis? What are you going to do for the next nine months? You can't stop taking the drug, even if you want to. To me, these dangers make the infusion approach a frighteningly bad choice.

An article in one medical journal delicately summed up things this way: "[T]he post-marketing experience with intravenous and, to a much lesser extent, oral bisphosphonates has raised concerns about potential side effects related to profound bone remodeling inhibition and osteonecrosis isolated to the jaws."

In 2011 this horrific side effect was even given its own acronym: BRONJ, for bisphosphonate-related osteonecrosis of the jaw.

Part of my concern about the bisphosphonate drugs is that because they are relatively new, there's still a lot that we really don't know about them. The long-term effects of bisphosphonates, in fact, are completely unknown.

It's worth keeping in mind that more than half of all serious adverse reactions are identified seven or more years after a drug receives approval from the Food and Drug Administration. What's more, the bisphosphonates were approved by the FDA after just three years of study, so as more people take the drugs for longer periods, I think we're likely to see additional adverse effects in the future.

We saw exactly this with estrogen replacement therapy, which before bisphosphonates came along was once the only FDA-approved osteoporosis medication. In time estrogen therapy was linked to uterine cancer, breast cancer, stroke, heart attacks, blood clots, and even dementia. Large studies showed that it did not enhance bone growth.

Even if you accept the many risks that go along with the bisphosphonate drugs, there's a much more important reason, in my judgment, to stay away from them: they don't really do what their manufacturers want us to believe they do.

Many women ask me if they need to be taking prescription drugs to strengthen their bones. My answer, nearly always, is no.

Some of them tell me that they have been diagnosed with osteopenia and are worried that it will develop into osteoporosis if they don't take the drugs. I know right then that I have a lot of educating to do — educating that a doctor really should do but that falls to me, as a consultant pharmacist, by default.

Osteopenia isn't a disease at all, although it sounds like one. It's nothing more than a classification that was developed by the

313

World Health Organization in the early 1990s to describe women whose T-scores from bone density scans are below peak level (that is, the average thirty-year-old woman's) but not the 2.5 or lower that would give them a diagnosis of osteoporosis. As you can imagine, a lot of women have T-scores that fall somewhere in this zone: about a third of all women fifty to sixty-four, and about two-thirds of those sixty-five and older. Many of these women are told they have osteopenia, without much in the way of explanation or additional information, and leave their doctor's office with a prescription for a bisphosphonate drug — this, too, without much in the way of explanation or additional information.

If they ask their doctor what osteopenia is, they're likely to be told that it's the medical term for pre-osteoporosis. That really doesn't help much either, as most women in this mile-wide category never go on to develop osteoporosis.

But the new classification of osteopenia has helped the manufacturers of bisphosphonate drugs to sell their products by getting doctors to prescribe them and by getting women to ask their doctors to prescribe them. The result is a market for bisphosphonates that's a much, much larger market than it should be.

Now it's time to look carefully at some of the numbers, which is exactly what the drug manufacturers don't want you to do.

When Merck, the manufacturer of Fosamax, says that the drug can reduce bone fractures by up to 50 percent in high-risk postmenopausal women, it's referring to a 2004 study that you would do well to read before you start taking a bisphosphonate. (Your doctor should have read the study but probably never bothered to do so.) Of the thousands of women in the study group (those with osteoporotic bone density and a history of previous fracture), 1.1 percent of those taking Fosamax experienced fractures, compared with 2.2 percent of those taking placebos (sugar pills). Because 1.1 percent is half of 2.2 percent, Merck is allowed to say that its drug reduces bone fractures by 50 percent.

As we've seen, relative risk reduction can sometimes be a useful tool for researchers. But it's not all that useful if you're trying to decide whether or not to take a prescription drug — especially, as with bisphosphonates, when the drugs are associated with some very serious and irreversible adverse effects.

In this case, for example, the relative risk reduction is 50 percent. The absolute risk

reduction — in my book, the most meaning-
ful statistic — is only 1.1 percent.

Think of it this way: if you had a 51
percent chance of developing osteoporosis
and a drug could reduce your risk to 49.9
percent, would you be eager to take that
drug? Probably not. Yet this is the same
absolute risk reduction that Fosamax, in the
key manufacturer-sponsored study, provided.

And remember that the study doesn't even
apply to women who aren't in the high-risk
group of postmenopausal women who have
already experienced fractures.

If you're not in this high-risk group, why
would you even think about taking a bisphosphonate drug? That's a good question
— and one that you ought to expect your
doctor to be able to answer.

Before you ask your doctor that question,
I'd recommend that you read — or at least
consult — a comprehensive report issued in
2004 by the Surgeon General of the United
States. It outlines the best ways to promote
bone health and prevent osteoporosis and
fracture, which is the goal that I always
focus on with my patients. I think that the
Surgeon General's advice is both sensible
and compelling. I'll summarize the main

approaches here.

Diet. Make sure that you're giving your bones the best chance to stay strong by getting enough calcium, vitamin D, and other bone-building nutrients.

In terms of bone health, not all calcium is created equal. A lot of the patients I see are taking some form of calcium carbonate — TUMS, Caltrate, and OsCal, for example — with the thought that it's good for their bones. I have to explain to them that what they're doing isn't helpful at all, as least as far as their bones (and probably even their stomachs) are concerned. Your body doesn't easily absorb calcium carbonate, which is really just chalk, especially as you grow older. What's more, because our body's pH level is self-adjusting, the constant ingestion of calcium carbonate can cause rebound acidosis, which can open the door to all kinds of bacterial infections (including *C. difficile* diarrhea and bacterial pneumonia, which are usually fatal in old people). In short, if you want to get calcium in your diet, you need to be taking calcium citrate (Citracal, for example), not calcium carbonate.

Vitamin D is required to help your system absorb calcium, to strengthen your bones.

The best way to get the vitamin D you need is by spending at least twenty minutes a day in sunlight. If you're not allowing your body to make enough vitamin D naturally, you probably should be taking something on the order of 2,000 IU of vitamin D_3 daily. If you avoid the sun, or don't know how much you need, a blood test called 25(OH)D will help you and your doctor determine how much supplemental vitamin D you need.

And here's the clincher: Some studies have shown that vitamin D is more effective in preventing fractures than are the bisphosphonate drugs. Some of my patients can't quite believe this when I tell them, but it's true. Sadly, however, our health care system isn't always based on science and common sense.

Exercise. Make sure that you exercise regularly. Weight-bearing exercise — walking, jogging, or anything else you can do on your feet — helps your bones stay strong, and strength training is just as important for your bones as it is for your muscles.

Reduce your risk of falls and fractures. You can trip over a vacuum cleaner when you're twenty and get back up with no harm done; you may not be so lucky when you're sixty-five. Because falls play a role in approximately 90 percent of all fractures, I advise my patients to take some simple and sensible steps at home to reduce their risk: things such as getting rid of throw rugs, adding some motion-activated lighting (especially in and around the bathrooms and stairs), and so forth. And I pay special attention to medications that may adversely affect balance and stability, including benzodiazepines, antihistamines, antidepressants, and antipsychotics. As the old saying goes, an ounce of prevention is worth a pound of cure — especially when the "cure" is a drug that brings with it lots of dangers.

It's important to remember that falls and the fractures that result from bisphosphonates — not "weak bones" — are what should concern you. And the things you can do to help prevent falls have benefits that go way beyond your bones. The bisphosphonate drugs, as we've seen, have no such benefits but have lots of drawbacks.

Assess your risks. "Women don't understand what their risk is, one way or the other," says Dr. Ethel Siris, the director of the Toni Stabile Osteoporosis Center at Columbia University Medical Center in

New York. I agree. So before you start on long-term drug therapy on the basis of a bone density scan, I'd recommend that you hit the pause button and ask your doctor for a real-risk workup.

Such a workup should take into account your age, weight, previous fracture history, family history, and other risk factors, which is far more useful from a predictive standpoint than a bone density scan. (A recent analysis of eleven separate studies, in fact, concluded that bone density scans "cannot identify individuals who will have a fracture.")

Suppose for a moment that you're a healthy fifty-year-old woman. Your doctor has just told you that you have osteopenia, based on a bone scan, and has recommended that you start taking a bisphosphonate. But did he or she also tell you that your actual risk for a hip fracture within the next ten years is less than 1 percent? Almost certainly not. And what would be your reason for taking the drug in the first place? Almost certainly, to avoid a hip fracture — the bone break we all fear the most. Hip fractures can have devastating consequences, including disability and death (15 to 20 percent of patients die within a year of the fracture).

But the truth is that hip fractures are a geriatric epidemic, not an epidemic among people in their fifties or sixties. According to a study published in the *Journal of the American Medical Association* in 2001, 81 percent of hip-fracture patients are seventy-five or older, and 43 percent are eighty-five or older. But the manufacturers of the bisphosphonate drugs aren't zeroing in on these age groups; they're targeting younger women who aren't even at risk.

Shockingly, neither the doctors who prescribe bisphosphonate drugs nor the companies that manufacture the drugs are in any position to say how long patients should be taking them. As the American College of Physicians puts it, "Evidence is insufficient to determine the appropriate duration of therapy."

Why would you start taking a drug if there is no scientific basis for knowing how long you should be on the drug? This is especially worrisome because of recent studies showing that the long-term use of bisphosphonates can actually *increase* the risk of stress fractures in the legs.

Let's return for a moment to the chemistry: by interfering with osteoclasts, the cells that clear out old bone, bisphosphonate drugs inhibit the process of resorption, with the result that old bone stays in place for much longer than would otherwise be the case. When someone first starts taking a bisphosphonate, the body keeps adding new bone cells but stops breaking down the old cells, which often makes for a dramatic difference in bone scan results.

After a year or so, however, the body's formation of new bone cells actually grinds to a halt. Scientists don't know why exactly, though it is clear that bisphosphonates also inhibit osteoblasts, our bone-building cells. Research by Joseph Lane, MD, the chief of the Metabolic Bone Disease Service at the Hospital for Special Surgery in New York, has found that while bisphosphonate drugs may be effective in slowing bone loss initially, their long-term use can actually diminish the quality of the bone.

In my work in nursing homes, I see, day after day, how the indiscriminate prescribing of bisphosphonate drugs can have horrific consequences, both for the patients who take them and for the Medicare system, which pays for them.

Several years ago, in reviewing the charts of patients at a combination nursing home and hospital, I noticed that eleven of them — all women, with an average age of eighty-six — were taking bisphosphonate drugs, as prescribed by a single doctor. Twice that year, I'd already recommended that the bisphosphonate therapy be stopped on each of these patients because of the serious problems with erosive esophagitis consistent with this age group as well as their lack of activity, impaired renal clearance, and overall deteriorating health. Now I saw that the doctor, in case after case, had rejected my recommendations.

"Patient stable at this time," he'd jotted on one of my recommendation forms. "I will decide on the treatment of the patient without your help," he'd written on another. Among his other notations: "No changes needed." "Patient old and needs to protect bones." "What do you have against helping old people?" "Drug salesman disagrees with your theory." "Let's wait and see."

By the end of the year, as it turned out, all eleven women had been admitted into the hospital section of the facility with erosive esophagitis and severe gastrointestinal bleeding, requiring many units of blood and intensive treatments. Nine of them returned to the nursing home section after treatment, but two didn't make it.

Since the nursing home and hospital are connected, I decided to go to the finance department of the facility to see how much it had cost to treat the eleven women. As I worked it out based on the facility's own records, the doctor's misguided insistence on prescribing bisphosphonates to these patients cost the health care system a total of slightly more than $1.2 million, or about $110,000 each, in addition to the two lives lost.

No price, of course, can be placed on that.

DOES DAD REALLY HAVE ALZHEIMER'S?: A LOOK AT DRUG-INDUCED DEMENTIA

We fear Alzheimer's disease more than we fear many other diseases because we don't know who it will attack or why, and we don't know how to treat it. Alzheimer's is an incurable, degenerative, and terminal disease that gradually robs those it afflicts of memory and mental capacity, and it doesn't stop until its victims forget how to breathe and die. This form of dementia was first described in 1906 by Alois Alzheimer, a German psychiatrist and neuropathologist, and in time the disease was named after him.

In the one-hundred-plus years since then, we really haven't made any substantial progress in diagnosing and treating the disease. There is no definitive test for Alzheimer's. No treatments to slow or stop the progression of the disease are, as of yet, available. The mean life expectancy following diagnosis is approximately seven years.

After death, in an autopsy, it is possible to examine the brain for the amyloid plaques and tangles that are thought to be the markers of Alzheimer's-type dementia and render, for the first time, something approaching a definitive diagnosis.

Many doctors are quick to label a patient exhibiting any kind of memory loss — or any form of cognitive impairment, really — as having Alzheimer's. The diagnosis is, by definition, subjective. If you frequently forget where you left your car keys, or what you watched on TV last night, or when you last ate dinner out in a restaurant, the specter of Alzheimer's disease will begin shadowing you, if only in the eyes of others, and only if you are, generally speaking, sixty or older.

Then there are the symptoms of advanced Alzheimer's, including confusion, irritability and aggression, mood swings, irrational behavior, more serious memory losses, and so on. Most of these are highly subjective too.

Every few months, a patient comes to me worried sick and frightened by the diagnosis of early-onset Alzheimer's just rendered by his or her doctor. But this same patient is nonetheless able to achieve a perfect score of 30 on the Mini-Mental State Exam

(MMSE), a questionnaire-type test that's used to screen for cognitive impairment. That's when it's time to start asking some serious questions about the drugs the person is taking.

Why? Many drugs can lead to a false-positive diagnosis for Alzheimer's disease. Tolterodine (Detrol), Pfizer's heavily promoted answer for what it has branded "overactive bladder," is a case in point. Since 1998, when Pfizer introduced the medication, there has been increasing evidence that Detrol and similar drugs that affect the activity of the brain chemical acetylcholine can impair cognitive function, especially in older people. So in addition to the more common adverse effects of dry mouth and constipation, medications such as Detrol and Oxybutynin (Ditropan) can cause confusion, disorientation, and hallucinations that resemble the symptoms of Alzheimer's.

Many, many other drugs bring about the same mental impairment. These include anticholinergic drugs alone or combined with other drugs for sleep; drugs for stomach disorders and high blood pressure; muscle relaxants; antianxiety pills; antiseizure medications; drugs for Parkinson's disease; statins; and a host of others. When older patients have just endured major surgery, health care practitioners know to expect days if not weeks or months of mental confusion as powerful anesthetics leave their bodies. Unfortunately, however, they often don't know how many prescription and over-the-counter medications can have exactly the same effect.

Drugs can cause dementia in two different ways. Many drugs, of course, affect the brain and central nervous system directly, causing a host of symptoms that fall in the Alzheimer's spectrum, including agitation, delirium, depression, dizziness, hallucinations, and memory loss. Other drugs can indirectly cause many of the same symptoms by producing conditions that are linked to dementia, like the accumulation of the drug in the body at toxic levels, the inability to metabolize the drug because of liver deficits consistent with age, and fluid and blood chemistry changes such as constipation, dehydration, low blood sugar, and urinary retention.

I often wonder how many people are diagnosed incorrectly with Alzheimer's disease because their doctors don't know or didn't question how many drugs — or drug combinations — can produce the same symptoms. My guess is that it's something like three out of four, but no one really knows. If it happens to you or someone you love, of course, that's all that matters.

I've never met Duane Graveline, MD, a former NASA astronaut and retired family physician, but his frightening experiences with two statin drugs show how close all of us can come to a mistaken diagnosis of dementia.

In 2000 Graveline was put on a low dose of the cholesterol-lowering drug atorvastatin (Lipitor) after his annual NASA physical at the Johnson Space Center in Houston showed an elevated cholesterol level.

About six weeks later, his wife found him circling aimlessly around their driveway and front yard. When she spoke to him, he didn't respond ("I didn't know who she was," Graveline recalled later), and it soon became clear to her that he had no recollection of recent events. He hesitantly consented to be driven to the hospital after a lot of coaxing by an old friend and fellow physician whom his wife had summoned.

Graveline's memory returned in about six hours, and a neurologist at the hospital rendered a diagnosis of transient global amnesia (TGA), "cause unknown." Graveline thought the cause might be the Lipitor — it was, after all, the only drug he was taking — but the doctors dismissed the suggestion. He stopped taking it anyway.

"But statins don't do that," was the response from each physician and pharmacist to whom he spoke.

A year later, the NASA doctors once again told Graveline that he needed to reduce his cholesterol and persuaded him to go back on Lipitor, this time at half the previous dose.

Six weeks later, Graveline landed in the hospital emergency room, having lost memory of everything in his life after high school. When he was told that he was a former astronaut and that he was married and had children, he laughed, finding the idea absurd. This time the amnesia lasted about twelve hours.

Again came the diagnosis of transient global amnesia, cause unknown. Graveline questioned the Lipitor connection even more emphatically but recalls hearing the same refrain from all of the doctors: "But statin drugs don't do that."

The former astronaut vowed never to take another statin drug. And, being a medical doctor, he also vowed to get to the bottom of what had happened to him. In time he learned of a study by Beatrice Golomb,

MD, an assistant professor of medicine at the University of California, that detailed cases similar to his own. "We have people who have lost thinking ability so rapidly," Golomb told a reporter in 2001, "that within the course of a couple of months, they went from being head of major divisions of companies to not being able to balance a checkbook."

The experience turned Graveline into a crusader against statin drugs, and over the years, he's received thousands of reports from people on cholesterol-lowering medications who refuse to believe that their episodes of confusion, disorientation, and forgetfulness are "senior moments" or the earliest possible signs of Alzheimer's disease. This one is typical:

My husband has been on Lipitor for several years, and I/we have noticed that more and more, his memory and focus have been impaired. We are told that there is no such evidence that Lipitor could cause this. I have watched my husband change from a Harvard Business School graduate who could accomplish more in four hours than most could in four days, to someone who has already had a TGA attack and, in the

two years since, has become more forgetful, is unable to complete tasks, loses
track of time — just about everything . . .
We know there is a problem and desper-
ately need help. Thank you.

The manufacturers of statin drugs dismiss
as "anecdotal" reports like the ones that
Graveline has collected. Not so easy to
dismiss are two double-blind, placebo-
controlled studies — the most scientifically
rigorous form of medical research — that
show cognitive impairment to be an adverse
effect of the cholesterol-lowering drugs
taken by some sixty million people in North
America.

Matthew Muldoon, MD, who led both
studies as an associate professor of medicine
at the University of Pittsburgh's School of
Medicine, concluded that cognitive impairment can be found in all people who take
statin drugs if sufficiently sensitive testing is
used.

"They are powerful drugs," he told an
interviewer in 2004. "We are obligated to
do more extensive research because we are
asking millions of people to take these drugs
for the rest of their lives."

I couldn't agree more, but I go a step
further with the older patients I see. Why

take such a big risk, I ask, for such a little benefit? And when it comes to drug-induced dementia, the risks are especially big.

When I started out in long-term care consulting more than forty years ago, I rarely saw or heard the word *Alzheimer's* used in clinical settings. Patients with dementia were labeled en masse as having "chronic brain syndrome" or "organic brain syndrome." It wasn't until the late 1970s and early 1980s that Alzheimer's disease, as a diagnosis, started appearing with any regularity.

Most of the time, patients with any form of dementia were given powerful antipsychotic drugs to subdue them and keep them from running away from the facility. The use of physical restraints was just as common as chemical restraints — antipsychotics, or neuroleptics, as well as all sorts of sedatives, hypnotics, and antidepressants. Nothing really seemed to work well, I came to realize, and I had serious problems with tying down human beings like wild animals to make them stay put. Often I saw the restraints cause bodily injuries. Just as troubling to me was what must have been going on in the minds of the people being sedated, subdued, and essentially straitjacketed.

I couldn't really fault the caregivers, though, because they had no idea how to care for this population of patients. Government regulations required that residents with dementia be subjected to something called "reality orientation" every day, a "therapy" that caused only more confusion, rage, and anguish. These residents were not in reality and weren't going to get there. Their minds were locked in time many years ago, and addressing *that* reality — not today's reality — was the key to dealing with them.

I noticed that patients with dementia were happier feeling that they were in control. If their reality at the moment was a picnic back in the 1950s, the best thing for the caregiver to do, I came to believe, was to have another piece of fried chicken and a spoonful of potato salad and tell the patient what a nice picnic it was.

Watching these patients and witnessing the degree of tranquility that could be achieved by seeing inside their reality made me realize that the existing acute-care procedures and customs had to be discarded, and palliative processes and procedures put in their place. When we shifted back in time by playing old music and showing old movies, our patients with dementia were clearly much happier and could let life go on by accepting themselves and their environment.

We also developed the idea of "bio boards." Each patient with dementia got a bulletin board with lots of memory-laden photos showcasing their families, friends, life achievements, and so forth. We used these bio boards to give names back to all of our patients and to develop plans of care consistent with their pasts. By allowing our patients to live freely in their own realities, we dramatically diminished the impulse to impose our reality on them with neuroleptics and other psychotropic drugs.

I remember one patient in the facility on high doses of three such drugs: haloperidol (Haldol), a neuroleptic; chlordiazepoxide (Librium), a benzodiazepine; and the sedative chloral hydrate. Nothing could make her quit screaming. I got up from my work area in the nursing station and asked one of the nurses to take me to the patient's room. There I saw the patient locked in a "geriatric chair": a chair on wheels with a tray to keep its occupant seated and in one place, like a baby's high chair. She was screaming and had a look of absolute horror on her face.

"We've tried everything," the nurse told me, "and nothing stops her from screaming all day and night."

I looked around her room and found the woman's bio board. I saw that she had been a beauty queen and had won the top title in her state in 1939. I picked up a hand mirror from the dresser, walked over to her, and held the mirror in front of her face. Immediately she stopped screaming, stared into the mirror, and started fixing her hair with her hands. So I left the facility and went to the local Kmart, where I bought a bunch of inexpensive children's makeup, some hair brushes, and a large mirror with a clip at the bottom.

I returned to the woman's room and clipped the big mirror on the tray attached to her Geri-Chair. Then I placed brushes, combs, lipstick, and other makeup in front of her. She quickly went to work fixing her face and hair. No screaming. I had put her back in her world, and she was perfectly happy to be there.

Over time we stopped all of the antipsychotics and hypnotics and started her on a mild dose of an antianxiety drug. The once-unstoppable screaming never returned, and the beauty queen seemed to be happy until the Alzheimer's disease finally took her life.

No reality orientation was needed, as she was real in *her* world and had never wanted to be in ours.

I remember another patient, dressed in a silk nightgown with matching silk slippers, who was restrained in a chair. A review of her meds showed that none of the drugs used to sedate her had been effective. She had bruises and cuts from trying to get out of the restraints. "Why is she restrained?" I asked. The nurse explained that the woman had been falling and that her family was afraid she would break a bone.

I wheeled the patient back to her room and discovered from her bio board that she had been the track-and-field coach at a local women's college for thirty-five years. Now she had Alzheimer's disease. I had the nurse call the woman's daughter and ask her to bring in a warm-up suit and her tennis shoes. The daughter did this reluctantly, explaining that "Mother always wore these" and that the family thought it would be nice for her to wear some prettier clothes. Nonetheless, on went the sweatpants, sweatshirt, white socks, and tennis shoes. "Let's untie her and see what happens," I said. The patient got up out of the chair, walked down the hall and around to the commons area, and sat down and started watching a Clark

Gable movie. The coach had returned, and she was happy to be home.

Back then patients would be admitted to the nursing home with no labs unless they had come from a hospital. The diagnosis listed by the patient's physician was taken at face value, and the treatment would be consistent with that diagnosis.

Something, I knew, was wrong. And so we set up a protocol of laboratory tests that would enable us to test the diagnosis and assumptions behind it by examining the patient and his or her chemistry. These labs often led to revelations about treatment.

For example, not long after we started this protocol, a man was admitted to the nursing home with a diagnosis of Alzheimer's disease. His labs showed that he had a TSH (thyroid-stimulating hormone) reading of 191. The average is around 2. This blood test revealed that he was severely hypothyroid, and from this we could be reasonably certain that his memory problems and maladaptive behavior were results of his thyroid gland not working properly. We immediately started levothyroxine therapy, and thirty days later, he was discharged, returning to live independently in his own home.

Over the years, I've found the laboratory reports to be absolutely invaluable in determining whether someone has been incorrectly diagnosed with Alzheimer's or some other form of dementia. Quite often I see nursing home patients who've just been admitted from a hospital and have Alzheimer's disease listed on their admitting data, but when I begin my medication review by reading the history and discharge report, I find that they've just had a hip replacement or some kind of traumatic surgery. Right then I know that in all likelihood they do not have Alzheimer's disease at all but are still experiencing significant cognitive impairment from the residual effects of the anesthesia, which may take two to three months to clear their bodies completely. Once it does, all the Alzheimer's-like symptoms go away.

When doing a comprehensive medication review for someone who's been diagnosed with Alzheimer's disease, I nearly always start by looking for drugs that should not or cannot be used in the very old. My short list includes beta-blockers, alpha-blockers, benzodiazepines, dopamine agonists, antipsychotics, tricyclic antidepressants, albuterol inhalers, anticholinergic agents, sedatives, hypnotics, sulfonylurea medications (used to treat diabetes), nitrofurantoins (used to treat urinary tract infections), statins, and any number of over-the-counter herbal drugs. (At the end of this chapter, you'll find an annotated version of the checklist that I use.)

I also look to see whether a Mini-Mental State Exam (MMSE) or other test was used to screen for cognitive impairment and what role it played in the diagnosis. All of these tests are highly subjective and, in my judgment, not all that useful as diagnostic tools, as they don't tell us much about what type of dementia a person has or what might be causing it. An MMSE or other screening test can't distinguish Alzheimer's-type dementia from drug-induced dementia, for example. What's more, test givers tend to see the scores through divergent lenses. While I may see a glass half full, so to speak, the next tester may see the glass half empty. Adding to the problem is that a lot may be riding on this very subjective numerical value, and patients, more often than not, know it. And so the clinician's approach to the test — how he or she explains it to the patient, as well as his or her interaction with the patient in administering it — has a lot to do with the results.

While I don't find the Mini-Mental State Exam all that useful from a diagnostic standpoint, I do find it useful in establishing a baseline against which I can evaluate the effects of changes in drug therapy. When we reach adulthood, our brain cells lose the ability to replicate (to divide and reproduce new cells, as happens elsewhere in the body). Therefore, if a patient's score improves from baseline with changes in his or her drug therapy, I have good reason to believe that the cognitive problems are drug induced and that further improvements are in store as we manage the medication end of his or her treatment more effectively. (And, of course, the reverse is true as well.)

These working tools typically help me determine whether medications might be causing the dementia or at least contributing to the degree of cognitive impairment. In such cases, relatively simple changes in drug therapy often improve the patient's quality of life dramatically. In older patients, nearly all the effects of drug therapy — good, bad, indifferent, and ugly — are related to body chemistry. In my view, this validates the need for regular laboratory tests (at least every six months, as a rule) when older people have health issues that could be caused by the medications they are taking.

In the case of Alzheimer's disease, there are a host of factors that have to be considered and ruled out before the patient is handed what invariably is a worrisome and life-changing diagnosis. Many times I see patients who for years have been treated with certain drugs said to be for Alzheimer's disease, and ultimately, I often find that it's the other drugs being taken by the patient that are causing the cognitive impairment.

Such cases particularly sadden and trouble me because most of the drugs used to treat Alzheimer's disease carry high risks that, in my judgment, plainly outweigh their possible benefits. Here the patients have been subjected to them for several years needlessly. I often wonder how many of them might not have lost so much of their lives if they had been able to see a consultant pharmacist before accepting the "fact" that they have Alzheimer's.

Not all cases can have happy endings, of course, but in my profession, there are few rewards greater than seeing a patient who was totally impaired from a cognitive standpoint on our initial visit drive himself or herself to see me for a follow-up visit.

■ ■ ■ ■

Any number of drugs and drug combinations can lead to false positives for Alzheimer's disease and other cognitive impairments. While most types of dementia cannot be reversed, drug-induced cognitive impairments can generally be reversed simply by stopping the offending drug (or drugs).

It's important to keep in mind that as you age, the adverse effects of any drugs you take will generally be more pronounced. They're also more likely to go undetected by doctors and other practitioners, who tend to attribute them to an underlying illness or simply to "old age," and that's especially true if they relate to memory or mental capacity.

Polypharmacy makes everything worse. A single medication may not trigger detectable cognitive impairment, but start pouring multiple medications into a patient's body — especially the anticholinergic drugs prescribed so commonly to older patients — and the cumulative impact can be both dramatic and dangerous.

Anticholinergic drugs work by blocking the neurotransmitter acetylcholine in the central and the peripheral nervous systems.

Acetylcholine is vital to a host of nervous system functions, so it's really not surprising that interfering with it can quickly cause some serious problems, including cognitive impairment, delirium, hallucinations, constipation, blurred vision, vertigo, dry mouth, reduced tear production, urinary retention, and prostate issues, among many others.

That's why anticholinergic drugs figure so prominently in my checklist of medications that can cause memory loss and other significant cognitive impairments.

So many drugs have anticholinergic properties that it would be nearly impossible to list them all. But as a shorthand approach, it's a good bet that any class of drug beginning with the prefix *anti* falls into this category, including antihistamines, antidepressants, antipsychotics, antispasmodics, antiparkinsonian drugs, and some antihypertensives.

Polypharmacy also makes the diagnostic equation far more difficult. The more complex a patient's medication mix, the more difficult it can be to tease out the specific drug or drugs that may be causing the cognitive impairment. What's more, the overall impairment may become more complex, too, as disorientation and memory loss enter the picture.

An additional roadblock, frequently, is that patients are so afraid of an Alzheimer's or dementia diagnosis that they don't share with their loved ones — or anyone else, for that matter — the problems they're experiencing. In these cases, unfortunately, there's no therapeutic intervention until the problems become glaringly obvious to others. Many times, if the patients had just been open about the problems they perceived from the outset, more could have been done and precious time saved.

Yet another diagnostic problem is that people do not readily think of most psychiatric symptoms as possible drug effects, and thus they are not likely to question whether those symptoms could be caused by the drugs that they — or a spouse or a parent — are taking. But my approach is always to think the other way around and, at least in older patients, to look at *every* psychiatric symptom as a possible side effect of a drug (or drugs).

Consider this list from the publication *Medical Letter on Drugs and Therapeutics* of psychiatric symptoms that can be drug induced: hallucinations, fearfulness, insomnia, paranoia, depression, delusions, bizarre behavior, agitation, anxiety, panic attacks, manic symptoms, hypomania, depersonalization, psychosis, schizophrenic episodes or relapses, aggressiveness, nightmares, vivid dreams, excitement, disinhibition, rage, hostility, mutism, hypersexuality, suicidality, crying, hyperactivity, euphoria, dysphoria, lethargy, seizures, Tourette's-like syndrome, obsessiveness, fear of imminent death, illusions, mood swings, sensory distortions, impulsivity, and irritability.

Add to that list other drug-induced symptoms that, while nonpsychiatric in nature, can nonetheless lead to cognitive impairment: delirium, confusion, disorientation, memory loss, amnesia, stupor, coma, and encephalopathy.

In short, there's often a lot to rule out before reaching the end point of a diagnosis of Alzheimer's disease.

If any symptoms of impaired memory or thinking arise, it's important that you and your physician — ideally, with the help of a consultant pharmacist — carefully review all of the medications you're taking, to determine if any of them might be the cause.

If the change in your mental condition was recent, you'll want to ask some basic questions: Was a drug recently added or stopped? Was one drug recently replaced with another? Were any dosages changed?

The need for an independent assessment

is very important in this review process because the physician (the probable prescriber of the drugs) often doesn't see problems, especially in older people, that the consultant pharmacist is trained to see.

Not long ago a patient came to me with severe memory problems, and he was visibly scared because his wife had died with Alzheimer's disease. He was in his eighties but still ran a small business and had gotten to where he couldn't remember his customers' names.

As I reviewed the seventeen different medications prescribed for him (all by the same physician), it became clear to me that the patient's memory problems were drug related and could easily be fixed. When the patient presented my report to his physician, the doctor became infuriated and told him that if he'd had problems with his medications he should have come to see him, not me. "But you ordered them," the patient replied, at which point the doctor told him that he wasn't interested in even looking at my report.

When the patient called me, I referred him to a physician with whom I enjoy a good working relationship. The changes were made, the patient's memory returned, and today he's happily running the business that he'd feared he might have to close.

DRUGS THAT CAN CAUSE COGNITIVE IMPAIRMENT: A PARTIAL CHECKLIST

- **Beta-blockers.** A class of drugs most often used to treat cardiac arrhythmias or hypertension, or to provide cardio-protection after a heart attack, beta-blockers diminish the effects of epi-nephrine (adrenaline) and other stress hormones. They cause many cognitive problems in older patients, including depression, anxiety, insomnia, confu-sion, and short-term memory loss. Some of the most commonly pre-scribed beta-blockers are metoprolol (Lopressor), atenolol (Tenormin), carvedilol (Coreg), sotalol (Betapace), bisoprolol (Zebeta), propranolol (Inderal), labetalol (Normodyne, Trandate), and nadolol (Corgard).
- **Benzodiazepines.** The first benzodi-azepine, chlordiazepoxide, was discov-ered by accident in 1955 and put on the market five years later as Librium. Another big-selling benzodiazepine, di-azepam (Valium), hit the market in 1963. Benzodiazepines are commonly prescribed for anxiety, insomnia, agita-tion, seizures, muscle spasms, and

alcohol withdrawal, and to sedate critically ill patients or those undergoing surgery. The chronic use of benzodiazepines heightens the risk of cognitive impairment, even in younger patients, and stopping them abruptly can trigger a withdrawal syndrome that includes sweating, agitation, confusion, hallucinations, and seizures. Once a patient reaches fifty or sixty years of age, though, any use of a benzodiazepine can be problematic, as changes in liver chemistry and renal function keep the drug from clearing the body. The residual concentration of the medication then climbs with each dose, leading to memory loss and multiple cognitive dysfunctions. That's why, in my judgment, benzodiazepines should never be used with older patients.

• **Narcotic agents.** Narcotics can cause delirium and are among the primary causes of postsurgery delirium, which is associated with longer hospitalizations, higher rates of nursing home placements, and higher in-hospital death rates. Meperidine (Demerol) is especially dangerous and has long been recognized as a drug that should not be given to older persons; it can cause confusion, disorientation, auditory and visual hallucinations, illusions, and persecutory delusions. Even tramadol (Rybix, Ryzolt, Ultram) can cause confusion.

• **Statins.** After muscle pain and weakness, cognitive problems are the second-most common side effect of Lipitor, Zocor, Pravachol, Mevacor, Crestor, and other cholesterol-lowering statin drugs. Hundreds of cases of statin-induced memory loss and transient global amnesia (TGA) have been reported to MedWatch, the FDA's safety information and adverse-event reporting program, and these undoubtedly are just a fraction of the total. Studies at the University of Alabama show that statin drugs inhibit the production of satellite cells, which are central to skeletal muscle regeneration and repair. This results in pains and cramps starting in the large leg muscles and working up the back, and is often the first sign of intolerance to the statin therapy. Patients who return to their physicians complaining of these symptoms often end up with a diagnosis of restless leg syndrome and a prescription for a dopamine agonist, which will only exacerbate the problems with memory and cognition. And then the drug cascade begins.

- **Tricyclic antidepressants.** The tricyclics, an older class of antidepressants also used to treat pain syndromes, are known to cause cognitive impairment. Because of the Beers criteria (see page 94), tricyclic antidepressants have the "Do Not Use" label in nursing homes, but other older patients are often subjected to them despite their serious adverse effects, which always follow — sometimes very quickly. Because of their anticholinergic properties, tricyclic antidepressants wreak havoc on all the involuntary muscle systems, causing, among other things, headaches, confusion, memory loss, delusions, hallucinations, and other serious cognition problems.

- **Anticonvulsants.** Anticonvulsants, originally used to treat epileptic seizures, and newer generations of these drugs have increasingly come to be used in the treatment of bipolar disorder, neuropathic pain, and muscle disorders associated with statin use.

Unfortunately, many anticonvulsants, by inhibiting the activities of neurotransmitters known as GABA (gamma-butyric acid) receptors in the central nervous system, can cause memory loss and dementia.

- **Muscle relaxants.** Because most muscle relaxants are anticholinergic, they mimic the tricyclic antidepressant drugs (see above) and cause the same cognitive problems of headaches, confusion, memory loss, delusions, and hallucinations. They should not be prescribed to older patients. Other muscle relaxant drugs, such as carisoprodol (Soma), act on the central nervous system and not on the muscles themselves. This CNS depression produces sedation and often alters the perception of pain. Insomnia, depression, memory loss, agitation, and psychological dependence are predictable adverse effects of carisoprodol.

- **Sleeping pills.** Sedative hypnotics such as benzodiazepines affect the central nervous system and can cause delirium. The most commonly prescribed sedatives are zolpidem (Ambien), temazepam (Restoril), and flurazepam (Dalmane). Sedative hypnotics should never be prescribed to geriatric patients, if only because they increase the risk of falls by 70 percent. Many health care professionals call Ambien "the amnesia drug," but all the sedative hypnotics can put an older patient on the road to cognitive impairment, especially because many doctors will treat his or her adverse effects with other drugs.

- **Corticosteroids.** Corticosteroids, which are frequently used to treat rheumatoid arthritis and many allergic reactions, are metabolized in the body to glucocorticoids, which are naturally occurring hormones that prevent or suppress inflammation and immune responses. For this reason, they can cause depression, anxiety, euphoria, personality changes, psychosis, and other mental changes. Corticosteroid therapy can also exacerbate mood swings and psychotic problems. There's another problem with corticosteroids. Geriatric patients who take them for long periods of time must be weaned off them very slowly to allow the body to start making glucocorticoids on its own. The failure to taper the geriatric patient off this class of drugs very slowly can be fatal.

- **Fluoroquinolone antibiotics.** These antibiotics, which are used to treat a variety of infections, are very popular, but, like almost all antibiotics, they can cause many serious adverse events in older patients with impaired renal function. Adding to the problem is that renal clearance in older patients can change very quickly, and if an infection is present, the clearance usually goes down. Excessive dosing of these antibiotics can cause agitation, anorexia, anxiety, ataxia, drowsiness, headache, insomnia, irritability, lethargy, light-headedness, malaise, nervousness, nightmares, paranoia, phobia, restlessness, vertigo, and delirium.

- **H_2 receptor antagonists and proton pump inhibitors (PPIs).** H_2 receptor antagonists are an older class of medications used to decrease stomach acid production. The first drug in this class was cimetidine (Tagamet). Because H_2 receptor antagonists are metabolized in the liver, extreme caution is warranted. When not dosed properly, they can cause agitation, confusion, delirium, hallucinations, hostility, paranoia, depression, and disorientation. Proton pump inhibitors (Prevacid, Prilosec, Nexium, and Protonix among them), a newer class of drugs that lower stomach acid, have pretty much taken the place of H_2 receptor antagonists. PPIs shut down several isozymes in the liver, which in turn makes the liver unable to metabolize many other drugs, rendering them ineffective. Consequently, many drugs then just pass through the body with no benefit, posing manifold risks to the patient. Because the PPI shifts the stomach's pH to a constant basic state, the stomach cannot then break down acid-sensitive drugs or food nutrients. With the absorption of B_{12}, folic acid, and many other vitamins blocked, patients typically develop anemia, which can lead to memory loss and dementia.

- **Antipsychotics.** These drugs, also called neuroleptics, are used to treat serious organic brain diseases such as schizophrenia and bipolar disorder. Older-generation ("typical") antipsychotics include chlorpromazine (Thorazine) and haloperidol (Haldol); newer-generation ("atypical") antipsychotics include risperidone (Risperdal), olanzapine (Zyprexa), quetiapine (Seroquel), and ziprasidone (Geodon). I see many patients who are prescribed these powerful drugs to treat their insomnia or anxiety. This is recklessly irresponsible. Antipsychotics can cause tardive dyskinesia and many other movement disorders, delirium, confusion, and depression, and even cardiac arrest and death. They were never designed to be used except in the appropriate treatment of psychotic disease.

- **Nitrates.** Nitrates, which are typically used to control angina (chest pain) or breathlessness in cardiac patients, can cause orthostatic hypotension (head rushes or dizziness after standing up) and syncope (loss of consciousness), which makes older patients especially feel out of mental control. Although this isn't memory loss, patients — and those around them — often perceive it to be.

- **Sulfonylurea derivatives.** This class of drugs has been used for more than fifty years to treat type 2 diabetes, a metabolic disorder with a high incidence among older adults. Because older diabetics nearly always have impaired renal clearance, sulfonylureas — used with or without metformin (Glucophage), another oral drug used to treat type 2 diabetes — can cause serious daily episodes of hypoglycemia, leading to falls, mental confusion, amnesia, and syncope.

Taking Charge: A Step-by-Step Guide to Controlling Your Medications (Rather Than Letting Them Control You)

Most of the patients I see in my office for an initial consultation have lost all control of their own health because they've lost all control of the medications they're taking. Fortunately, they sense that something is wrong and that the medications they're taking may be doing more harm than good. Sometimes, of course, it's a spouse or family member who sees most clearly that the medications have made things worse and decides to seek out the help of a specialist like me. And occasionally doctors send their patients to me because they realize that a specialist in pharmacotherapy may pick up things that they're not really trained to see.

I'm nearly always amazed, too, at how little the patients I see for the first time know about the medications they're taking. When I ask, "Do you know why you're taking this medication?" or "Do you know why your doctor prescribed this?" the answer, with alarming frequency, is "No," "I don't know," "I'm not sure," or something along those lines. When I ask patients why they are taking so many different medications for high blood pressure, only rarely can they offer any kind of answer. The same generally goes for questions such as "Do you know why your doctor put you on this diabetes drug?" or "Do you know that someone your age shouldn't be taking this medication?" or "Do you know that this drug could be causing some of the symptoms you're experiencing?"

I think of the patients who spend untold hours managing their investments or finances, pursuing hobbies and other recreational activities, traveling to see their children and grandchildren, and so forth. But somehow they don't see fit to do the same when it comes to understanding and managing the medications they're taking.

It's not just about your health, it's about your pocketbook. You can be wasting many thousands of dollars a year by taking drugs that don't work, drugs with risks that outweigh their potential benefits, multiple drugs for the same illness or condition, expensive drugs with less costly but equally effective counterparts, drugs that your body can't adequately absorb, drugs to deal with adverse effects caused by other drugs, drugs to treat conditions that can be treated just as well with nondrug therapies, and so on.

If you're taking lots of drugs, a "medication audit" may help you save lots of money. Here are a few examples of what I mean:

- *You're taking different forms of the same drug.* I once saw a patient who'd been prescribed Prinivil, Vasotec, and Zestril — three different ACE inhibitors — at the same time.
- *You're taking a drug with no established therapeutic benefit.* If your doctor advised you to take a statin merely because your cholesterol is high, you're probably wasting your money.
- *You're taking a drug that's not doing what it's supposed to do.* If you're taking a medication for your diabetes and your blood sugar values are still too high, your doctor probably needs to try a different drug.

There is a lot, though, that you can and should do on your own. The step-by-step guide that follows will help put you in control of all the medications you're taking, help you avoid dangerous medication errors, and, in so doing, put you on the road

360

to better health.

What's more, the hours you invest at the front end will be repaid many times over in your journeys through the health care system. You'll begin to see the benefits right away — like the next time you visit a new doctor, for example, and are asked to fill out a patient information form.

I can assure you, too, that the mere process of taking charge of your medication regimen will leave you feeling a whole lot better.

Compile a "personal medication dossier" and always keep it up to date. This is basically an annotated list that will help you and members of your family keep track of every medication you take to keep yourself healthy. Having all of this information in an easily accessible form also will help your doctor, pharmacist, hospital, and other health care professionals take better care of you.

Begin by making a detailed, up-to-date list of all the prescription medications that you take, being sure to include any that you use in nonpill form (liquids, drops, ointments, and so forth). Next, do the same for all your nonprescription medications, even those that you use only occasionally. Finally, add any dietary supplements that you take — products that supply vitamins, minerals, fatty acids, fiber — as well as herbal remedies, laxatives, and foods consumed for therapeutic reasons.

Include the following information for each medication and other products on the list:

- The name of the drug or other product, including, where applicable, the generic name, brand name, and dosage form (for instance, acetaminophen/ Tylenol 500 mg, and so on).
- What it looks like (round blue tablet, white-and-red capsule, clear liquid), including the imprint on each tablet or capsule.
- How much you take (1 tablet, 1 teaspoon, 2 drops, and so on).
- How you take it (by mouth, with food, by injection).
- When you are supposed to take it (three times a day, at lunchtime, before you go to bed).
- Special instructions for taking it (on an empty stomach, with a glass of water, sitting up for at least thirty minutes afterward).
- When you started taking it.
- When you expect to stop taking it.

- Why you take it (for arthritis, for blood pressure, to lower cholesterol).
- Who recommended that you use it (family doctor, cardiologist, nutritionist, self).

Finally, make another list that includes current contact information — names, addresses, telephone and fax numbers, e-mail addresses, and so forth — for all the physicians and other health care professionals you see or have seen and for any pharmacies that fill prescriptions for you.

If you don't know why you're taking any of the medications or other products on the list, ask. Contact the physician or other health care professional who instructed or advised you to take it and add that information to your list.

If you're taking more than one medication for the same problem or medical condition, ask the physician who prescribed them to explain why. This is especially important if more than one physician you've seen has prescribed medications to treat the same problem — high blood pressure, say, or joint pain.

Physicians are sometimes reluctant to

discontinue a medication that another physician has prescribed, so you need to be sure that drugs are not just being piled on top of one another. For example, I've seen patients who are taking five or six different blood pressure medications when a sound rule of practice is to prescribe no more than two.

If you are taking medications that were prescribed by doctors you do not see on a regular basis, or no longer see at all, ask your primary care physician whether you still need to be taking them. Whenever you see a new doctor — whether it's because you've moved or switched insurance plans, for example, or because of a change in your health — you should make sure that the prescriptions from the doctor you've left don't become your excess pharmaceutical baggage. This is especially important with "lifetime drugs" such as insulin, thyroid products, statins, heart medications, and immunosuppressants.

Share your medication dossier with all the doctors and other health care professionals you see and bring a copy with you to every office visit. It's important to remember that one physician's records may not reflect all the medications you've been taking, especially if you use a lot of over-the-counter products and see other practitioners with whom your doctor is not in regular contact.

Providing your complete medication picture to everyone who treats you is a big step toward making sure that you get the best care possible.

Whenever a doctor writes you a prescription, look at it before you leave the office and make sure not only that you understand it but also that it matches what the doctor told you. If knowledge is power, leaving a doctor's office with a little slip of paper that you can't even read instantly puts you in the danger zone. So if there's anything you don't understand or anything that isn't clear, ask for an answer or clarification before you leave the office.

I also advise my patients to do the following:

First, make sure that the prescription is written clearly and in plain English. As a pharmacist, I know that *bid* means "twice a day" and that *hs* means "at bedtime," but you probably don't. (Doctors use abbreviations based on Latin words to tell your pharmacist how to fill the prescription as well as how they want you to take the medication.) And if you can't read your doctor's handwriting, your pharmacist might not be able to, either.

So don't settle for a scribbled prescription that consists mostly of abbreviations you can't understand. Politely ask your doctor to write out the prescription in a form clear enough for you to read and understand; then ask him or her to read it aloud as you're both looking at it. This way, you'll dramatically minimize the chances of something getting lost in translation.

Second, as a safety measure, ask your physician to include both the generic name and the brand name (if applicable) of the medication on the prescription form.

Third, ask your doctor to write the purpose of the medication on the prescription form. That will also help reduce the risk of a mistake, as it provides another checkpoint for the pharmacist in cases where drugs have very similar names — like Fosamax, a bisphosphonate drug used to treat osteoporosis, and Flomax, a drug used to treat benign prostatic hyperplasia (an enlarged prostate) in men.

Whenever a doctor writes (or offers to

write) you a prescription, especially for a condition such as inflammation or pain, ask whether it might make sense to try a nondrug approach first and also what the consequences of going without the drug might be. Don't be afraid to ask your doctor these kinds of "What if?" questions. There are lots of reasons why this makes sense.

Take the relatively common conditions of tennis elbow (lateral epicondylitis) and golfer's elbow (medial epicondylitis). If you see your doctor or orthopedist for either condition, you're likely to come away with a prescription for an NSAID (nonsteroidal anti-inflammatory drug) or a corticosteroid injection. Yet these interventions, studies show, generally are no better than rest, exercise, and physical therapy, and they both come with their own — and not insubstantial — risks.

Or take depression, which affects nearly all of us at one time or another. Depression is an episodic illness that's sometimes precipitated by events such as a death in the family, going through a divorce, or losing your job. An episodic illness comes and goes, and some people see their depression lift and never come back. A recent study, based on data submitted to the Food and

Drug Administration by the manufacturers of three widely prescribed antidepressants — fluoxetine (Prozac), paroxetine (Paxil), and venlafaxine (Effexor) — concluded that they work no better than placebo for most patients who take them. (Predictably, an official of the American Psychiatric Association criticized the study by saying that doctors typically need to try three different antidepressants before they "find the one that works for a particular individual.")

Finally, when a doctor suggests that you take a new prescription drug as preventive therapy (for high blood pressure or high cholesterol, for example), don't forget to ask about the all-important NNT (number needed to treat). If your doctor doesn't know the NNT associated with the drug and declines to look it up for you, take that as a sign that he or she may not know all that much about the drug in question.

With every new prescription, make sure that your doctor explains exactly what the medication is supposed to do and how long it will take for it to work. If your doctor doesn't explain this to you, ask bluntly, "When should I expect the medicine to begin to work, and how will I know if it is working?"

These are extremely important questions; otherwise you might not know whether or when, after taking a medication, you should get back in touch with your doctor.

Part of this discussion with your physician should involve the expected duration of treatment and how refills of the medication, if any, will be handled.

With every new prescription, make sure that your doctor explains possible adverse effects or events to you in terms that you can understand. Your doctor is supposed to be the expert, so don't settle for buck-passing ("I've never had any problems with this drug" or "You'll get a sheet at the pharmacy that explains them"). You want to leave your doctor's office with answers to these questions:

- What are the medication's possible side effects, and what do I do if they occur?
- Will this medication work safely with the other medications — prescription and nonprescription — that I am taking? If you've brought along your dossier, you'll be able to ask simply, "Will this medication work safely with all the other medications on this list?"

- Will this medication work safely with the dietary or herbal supplements that I am taking?
- What food, drink, or activities should I avoid while taking this medicine?

If your doctor gives you samples of a medication, ask him or her to check to make sure that it can be safely taken with your other medications. Most pharmacies use computer-based systems to check for drug interactions and allergies; chances are that your doctor doesn't have something like that. Dispensing samples bypasses this important checkpoint.

If possible, buy all your medications at one location. That location should preferably be a pharmacy with a reputation for personalized services and with a computer program that can monitor your prescription history for duplications and interactions. If the pharmacy you use doesn't fit into that category, consider switching to one that does.

Before filling a prescription, make a copy of the form or ask the pharmacy to make a copy for you. Otherwise, once you hand over your prescription at the pharmacy, you'll no longer have a record of what your doctor prescribed. This way, you'll have the information in hand to help resolve any questions about whether you got the right medication.

A study by the Massachusetts College of Pharmacy and Allied Health Sciences found that 88 percent of all medication errors involved the wrong drug or the wrong dose.

Whenever you have a prescription filled, ask the pharmacist to go over the dosing and instructions with you. Make sure they match what you were told in the doctor's office and what's on the label. If they don't, ask the pharmacist why — and, if need be, ask him or her to get in touch with your doctor's office for clarification.

When it comes to medications, there's no such thing as a stupid question. For example, does "three times daily" mean taking a dose around the clock at precise eight-hour intervals or just spaced out during your regular waking hours? There's only one way to be sure, and that's to ask.

And don't forget to check the basics: that it's your name on the label, and that it's your prescription. If you're handed a stapled-up paper bag with the prescription inside, open the bag while you're still at the prescription counter and make sure that you're getting exactly what you think you're supposed to be getting. Mistakes, as the saying goes, do happen.

Of the three billion or so prescriptions filled each year at neighborhood pharmacies, according to the National Patient Safety Foundation, mistakes are made in about thirty million. You don't want yours to be one of them.

Before you leave the pharmacy, it's not a bad idea to open up the container and verify, with the pharmacist's help, that you actually got the medication you were prescribed. This is especially important if your prescription was filled by a pharmacy assistant or technician.

Whenever you have a prescription refilled, look at the medication before you leave the pharmacy to make sure that it's the same medication you've been taking. Are the tablets or capsules the same color, size, and shape as the ones you've received in the past? If the medication comes in the manufacturer's packaging, is the packaging the same? If anything about the medication seems different to you, ask the pharmacist about it.

■ ■ ■ ■

Carefully read the package insert that comes with any medication you use, along with any additional information that the pharmacy provides. Spending just a few minutes reading this material could alert you to something you or the doctor overlooked.

Tell your doctor immediately about any problems you are having with your medications, including anything you suspect could be an allergic reaction or other side effect. If you start feeling worse, call your doctor's office immediately. The same is true if the medication doesn't seem to be working.

Take all medications exactly as directed. Before you use any medication, you should know when to use it, how much to use, and for how long to use it. If you find yourself unable to understand the directions for any medication, call the doctor or pharmacist before using it.

Don't chew, crush, or break any capsules or tablets unless instructed to do so. Some extended-release medications are absorbed too quickly when chewed, for example, which could be unsafe. Others have enteric or "gastro-resistant" coatings designed to release the drug only when it reaches the intestines.

Don't try to change the dosing yourself. "Doubling up" the dose of a medication because you think it's not working the way it should is one of the most dangerous things you can do; so is supplementing a prescription drug with over-the-counter medications.

And be sure to read the medication's label every time you use it, and never take medication when you're not fully awake. You could find yourself putting drops intended for your ears into your eyes or mistakenly taking someone else's medication.

Store all your medications exactly as directed. Some medications need to be refrigerated, while others can't be exposed to extreme temperatures. And it's not a good idea to store medications in the bathroom medicine cabinet or in direct sunlight. Humidity, heat, and light can affect their potency and safety.

Keep all your medications in their original containers. That way, you can be sure which is which and how to take them.

■ ■ ■ ■

Have your medications reviewed by a consultant pharmacist at least once a year, and more often if you think your medications are not doing what they're supposed to do or are having unintended consequences.

I recommend that you find a board-certified geriatric pharmacist who works with individual patients. (Many are employed by universities, hospitals, and other institutions and do not provide one-on-one consultations.) The Commission for Certification in Geriatric Pharmacy (www.ccgp.org) offers a state-by-state lookup tool to help you find such a pharmacist near you. You can find more information about the CCGP in the resources section of this book on page 411.

I ask new patients to "brown-bag" all of their prescription and over-the-counter medications. That way I can see exactly what they've been taking and ask better questions.

Share a copy of your medication dossier with a family member or friend, or at least let them know where you keep

it. That way, in an emergency, your family member or friend will be able to help minimize the chances of medication errors by the medical team that's taking care of you.

While all this may seem like a lot of work, there are some free tools that can make everything easier.

If you're a pen-and-paper kind of person, a good starting point could be My Medicine List, a form created by the American Society of Health-System Pharmacists to help you keep track of everything you take. You can download a PDF copy at www.safemedica tion.com and fill it out by hand; you can also fill out the form on your computer, save it that way, and print out a copy. It's also available in Spanish.

If you use a smartphone, a growing number of applications (apps) are available to help you track the medications you're taking. Some allow you to enter your prescription information merely by scanning a QR code — the blobby Quick Response bar code that's on an ever-growing number of packages — into your phone. Some will tell you which of your prescriptions are coming up for refills. Some remind you when you need to take medications.

My favorite, though, is My Medication Tracker, which was created by *Consumer Reports* with funding from the National Library of Medicine of the National Institutes of Health. You can use it on your home computer to maintain a complete, up-to-date list of all the medications you take, including dosages, expiration dates, how much you paid for each medication, directions on how to take your medicines, and the number of refills left. You can also record and store information about your medical conditions, vaccinations, allergies, and insurance coverage.

PRESCRIPTION FOR CHANGE: HOW TO FIX A BROKEN HEALTH CARE SYSTEM

A couple of months ago, I had a colonoscopy, as I do at five-year intervals, and because of a dip in my iron stores that was detected at the time, the doctor ordered an upper GI endoscopy. Although Medicare and my Medigap policy paid the claims for both procedures, copies of the bills were sent to me. They offered a dramatic snapshot of what's so horribly wrong with our health care system.

The bills for the two procedures added up to more than $8,000, and the physician fees pushed the total to more than $10,000. Keep in mind that these are two fairly straightforward diagnostic procedures. Now, I'm just one of the 47 million or so Medicare beneficiaries nationwide, including nearly 1.3 million in my home state of Georgia, but I don't even have to do the math — and you probably don't, either — to understand why Medicare is on a financially untenable path. Something has to be done to make costs appropriate to services, and it has to be done before the baby boomers all get on board with us.

Starting in 2011, Medicare began covering screening tests for colorectal cancer — including colonoscopies, sigmoidoscopies, and fecal occult blood tests — at no charge to beneficiaries. This is a good thing, as these are among the best preventive health care measures we have, and more Americans need to have them. But in our nation's upside-down health care system, they cost — or at least are billed at — way more than they ought to be.

As I see it, the approaches that most politicians advance to curb the nation's runaway spending on health care aren't in any way going to work to save the system — or save us. The savings have to be generated from the bottom up, not from the top down. The present system of setting fees from the top down hasn't worked, is out of control, and delivers lower-quality health care.

I often hear people say that we, as Americans, have "the best medical care in the world," or "the best health care system in the world." But the truth is, we don't. If you look at two of the most basic statistical yardsticks — infant mortality and life expectancy — the United States falls in the bottom fourth of the world's industrialized countries. The rest of the leading indicators, to borrow a term from economists, are something of a mixed bag. The United States does well in some areas, such as cancer care, and not so well in others — particularly those where better prevention and treatment could dramatically reduce mortality rates. An ounce of prevention really is worth a pound of cure, but our health care system just doesn't deliver it.

In my day-to-day work, I also hear more complaints than you can possibly imagine about doctors and the way health care is delivered. My sample is biased, of course, because people typically come to me after they've lost faith in those who are treating them, or at least in the therapies those who are treating them have put in place. But it's always striking to me how these people never talk about how we have "the best health care system in the world," and I don't think I've ever heard that sentiment expressed seriously in a nursing home or similar facility. The disconnect is extreme.

A few years back, I was fascinated to read a survey of primary care physicians in five countries. It found the practices of physicians in the United States to be more limited in knowledge, to provide less patient access outside of traditional working hours, and to be among the least likely to work in teams. Here, too, the disconnect is extreme.

I first started working as a consultant pharmacist at about the time that Title 18 and Title 19 of the Social Security Act were enacted in 1965. Title 18 ("Health Insurance for the Aged and Disabled") is known as Medicare, and Title 19 ("Grants to States for Medical Assistance Programs") is known as Medicaid. I had the sense from nearly the beginning that both of these programs were fundamentally skewed away from patient care.

In the realm of pharmacy, for example, the federal government set the prices that a pharmacist could charge for each prescription, set the prices that a nursing home could charge, and so on down the line with other health care professionals. But it didn't place a ceiling on what the pharmaceutical industry could charge for each drug. I knew then that this would be an open door to trouble, and it's turned out to be exactly that.

I was looking the other day at Donnatal, a propriety combination medication for the treatment of intestinal cramping. Donnatal was around in 1965 and used extensively. The cost to the pharmacist back then was $12 per one thousand tablets. The pharmacist would package the tablets for the patient in the quantity specified by the doctor with a professional charge of $1.65 per prescription. Today the federal government pays $4.25 per prescription, but the cost to the pharmacist is $600 per one thousand tablets. If you wonder why there are runaway costs in the Medicare and Medicaid programs, this isn't a bad place to start.

The Medicare and Medicaid programs also put into place the requirement that a consultant pharmacist visit every nursing home on a monthly basis, review the drug therapy of each resident receiving skilled care, and report any contraindicated, otherwise inappropriate, or ineffective medications to the prescribing physician for changes. Back then, a local retail pharmacy would provide the drugs to the nursing home residents and also provide the consulting services. One problem with this arrangement, however, was that while the local retail pharmacist could make money providing the drugs, he or she wasn't really trained in the clinical aspects of performing drug therapy reviews.

In 1974, recognizing that consultant

pharmacists were significantly improving patient care in the nation's nursing homes, the federal government extended their responsibilities to cover all residents — not just those receiving skilled care. (Before then, registered nurses were allowed to do the drug therapy reviews for residents in intermediate care.) This change at the federal level made many retail pharmacists even more reluctant to provide consultant services. It was at right around this time that I decided to work exclusively as a consultant pharmacist. To me, putting retail pharmacists in charge of reviewing the drugs they provided to nursing homes posed obvious conflicts of interest. The consultant pharmacist, as I saw it, needed to be totally independent. As it turned out, retail pharmacists in my area were only too happy to let me fill the consulting role while they continued providing the drugs.

I had no financial ties to either the nursing homes or to the retail pharmacists, which gave me complete freedom in suggesting ways to improve the drug therapy management of patients and to enhance patient care. I still, of course, had doctors to contend with, and often their egos — and insecurities from having their decisions reviewed and sometimes questioned —

made for a difficult work environment.

At the same time, the big pharmacy companies and corporate nursing home chains, seeing a way to make huge profits in this environment, started buying out small pharmacies throughout the United States and taking over the business of providing drugs to nursing homes. These big corporate operations aimed to place their own consultant pharmacists in nursing homes as a means of getting drugs changed to their formularies, having made special deals with the major drug manufacturers. To do this, they'd often offer their consultant-pharmacist services for nothing or next to nothing, or offer cash rewards to get their foot in the nursing home's door, and then make up for it by dispensing an ever-increasing volume of drugs. Thus, in these cases, the consultant pharmacists would be working to increase the number of drugs prescribed rather than to reduce them.

The federal government mostly turned a blind eye to these unethical practices, and multitudes of dedicated independent consultant pharmacists dropped out of the picture. The consultant pharmacists working for these large corporate operations, meanwhile, were assigned unrealistically large patient loads, making it impossible for them to perform comprehensive drug reviews. Many were instructed to advise doctors to switch to the brands of drugs in the corporate formulary or to add additional drugs to the regimen as a means of boosting profits. They even pressured the consultant pharmacists to go along by making the quantity of drugs they moved part of their job evaluations.

A few years back, when I was serving as an adviser to the governor of Georgia on a committee seeking to reduce the cost of the state's Medicaid program, I had an opportunity to see, in very stark terms, just how much the system has been gamed. I compared the drug cost per patient per day — a standard measure in our industry — for consultant pharmacists in different categories. For the independents, the average was $8.50 a day. For the "corporates," with their own consultant pharmacists, the average was $18 a day. For the consultant pharmacists employed directly by the big nursing home chains, the average was $25 a day.

To me, the conclusion was clear: the consultant pharmacists employed or retained by drug sellers — the corporate and nursing home pharmacies — were not really doing their job at all. Under their supervision, more and more drugs were being ordered for patients, and more and more patients were being overmedicated in the name of corporate greed. And all this was going on with little in the way of real checks and balances in the system, either from a health care standpoint or from a financial standpoint.

In 2005 the federal government accused PharMerica, a corporate provider of pharmacy services to long-term care facilities, of violating federal antikickback laws by paying $7.2 million for a small Virginia pharmacy with "virtually no operating history" in exchange for a commitment from the seller — who owned seventeen nursing homes and eight assisted-living facilities — to send all of its Medicare and Medicaid pharmacy business to PharMerica for seven years. After being threatened with more than $21 million in fines and damages and a ten-year ban on participating in any federal health care programs, PharMerica agreed to pay just under $6 million to settle the case.

And in 2009 the federal government announced that Omnicare, the largest pharmacy in the nation that specializes in providing drugs to nursing home patients, had agreed to pay $98 million to settle charges that it had solicited or paid a variety of kickbacks. Omnicare was alleged to have paid kickbacks to two large nursing home chains in exchange for pharmacy-services contracts, for example, and to have solicited and received kickbacks from the pharmaceutical manufacturer Johnson & Johnson in exchange for agreeing to have its consultant pharmacists recommend that physicians prescribe Risperdal, an antipsychotic drug manufactured by Johnson & Johnson, to nursing home residents. Johnson & Johnson's kickbacks to Omnicare allegedly took a variety of forms, including rebates for participation in its "Active Intervention Program" for Risperdal and payments disguised as data purchase fees, educational grants, and fees to attend Omnicare meetings.

The federal government further alleged that Omnicare regularly paid kickbacks to nursing homes by providing consultant-pharmacist services at below-market rates — below the company's cost, in fact — to induce them to use Omnicare for pharmacy services.

"These defendants broke the law to take advantage of our nation's most vulnerable citizens — the elderly and the poor," Tony West, the US assistant attorney general who heads the Justice Department's Civil Division, said in announcing the settlement. "Illegal conduct like this can undermine the medical judgments of health care professionals, lead to patients being prescribed medications they do not need, and drive up the costs of health care."

Unfortunately, the PharMerica and Omnicare cases haven't yet led to real reform of the system.

Over the years, I've had many consultant pharmacists call me to complain about the system and to advise them on what they should do. That's easy, I would say in so many words: quit. I'd explain that you can't allow others to dictate how you practice your profession. The world being what it is, though, most people won't let a principle get in the way of a paycheck. But I've always thought that if your boss is doing wrong, it's best to get out of the picture, and the sooner the better.

The way I see it, the big corporate operations have set back my profession many years by not allowing the consultant pharmacists who work for them to carry out the valuable drug therapy management that the American Society of Consultant Pharmacists fought so hard to put into place. The federal government's overall monitoring of the system has been pitifully deficient. The regulations that implemented the 1987 Nursing Home Reform Act — the law that established the rights of residents and quality standards for nursing homes nationwide — required the consultant pharmacist to make suggestions in writing to the physician about drug therapy management issues. The physician then had the right to accept or reject a suggestion, but if rejected, the physician was required to record his or her reasons for not following the pharmacist's suggestion. This regulation was an excellent way to have doctors document the rationale for the use of any given drug.

The American Medical Association and similar organizations — many of whose members chafe at the idea of anyone else questioning or challenging their prescribing habits — have fought hard to have this portion of the regulation removed. Although the AMA's campaign failed, and the regulation is still in place, most doctors no longer explain why they're rejecting the consultant pharmacist's suggestion. As I see it, this has pretty much stopped the huge progress being made in improving health care through comprehensive drug therapy management.

As long as the regulations go unenforced

and physicians are allowed to reject drug therapy recommendations without explanation, it doesn't seem to me that there can be much improvement in the system. As it stands now, even if a consultant pharmacist identifies a serious medication problem, the doctor doesn't have to change it or even explain why. This comes at a tremendous cost to the health care system, and the cost goes much further than what's paid for the drugs. To get the whole picture, you need to include the extra costs of emergency room visits, hospital admissions, extensive (and expensive) tests and lab work, nursing costs, and on and on and on.

Congress did a good thing in 2001 by deciding to subsidize the costs of prescription drugs for Medicare beneficiaries. The devil, as the saying goes, was in the details. The Centers for Medicare and Medicaid Services (CMS), in writing regulations to implement Medicare Part D, added something called "medication therapy management" but then proceeded to delegate this important job to the insurance companies that participate in the program. The insurance companies often delegate this important job to technicians who sit behind computer screens looking at general practice guidelines for the use of particular drugs. It's cookbook medicine at its worst.

Here's an example from my case files. I recently suggested the use of venlafaxine (Effexor) ER, an extended-release serotonin-norepinephrine reuptake inhibitor (SNRI) that's used to treat depression and anxiety, to help move an older patient, through a slow tapering, off a powerful antipsychotic. The insurance company refused, suggesting that the doctor use sertraline (Zoloft), paroxetin (Paxil), fluoxetine (Prozac), or citalopram (Celexa) instead. This astounded me, because none of these drugs is an appropriate substitute for venlafaxine. They're all older-generation selective serotonin reuptake inhibitors (SSRIs) that do not have any antianxiety properties. And they were inappropriate in this case for two reasons: older patients lack the hepatic enzymes needed to metabolize SSRIs properly, and all SSRIs have a higher adverse-event profile than is desirable. Venlafaxine is a geriatric-friendly drug with a lower adverse-event profile. The cookbook-medicine approach in this case not only prolonged the patient's suffering but also caused the health care system to spend about four times the amount of money that it should have.

Here's another example. Recently the medical director of one of the nursing homes I work in showed me a copy of a letter that he'd received from a medication therapy management firm in Florida. The letter pointed out that Alice Jones, one of the nursing home's residents, had been diagnosed with type 2 diabetes but hadn't been prescribed an ACE inhibitor to protect her kidneys. I called the firm and asked to speak to a pharmacist who could explain the reasoning in the letter. The pharmacist explained matter-of-factly that, according to the relevant practice guidelines, anyone with type 2 diabetes should be on an ACE inhibitor for kidney protection.

"Do you know anything about Ms. Jones?" I asked, knowing that the answer would be no. "Well," I explained, "she's an eighty-seven-year-old African American with a renal clearance of twenty cubic centimeters a minute, which makes the drug you want to put her on contraindicated." (ACE inhibitors don't work in African Americans and also require a renal clearance of at least 30 cc/min.) I went on to point out that there is no kidney protection from this drug or any drug at age eighty-seven but that there *are* serious and possibly fatal adverse events. The pharmacist asked to put me on hold and never came back on the line.

The point is, you can't do effective drug therapy management unless you have the patient in front of you, are able to ask questions and sometimes administer simple tests, and have access to the last six to twelve months of laboratory tests. Only then can you adequately evaluate the patient's conditions and existing drug therapy and come up with fact-based recommendations to improve the patient's life. You can't do this by telephone or by sending out letters generated by a computer program.

It takes two to three hours, as a rule, to do all this conscientiously — that is, in a way that's worth something to the patient or to the third-party payer. That's why CMS should allow insurance companies to do what they do best, and why CMS should contract independently with consultant pharmacists to conduct drug therapy management reviews under an appropriate fee schedule. I think CMS would quickly realize two to four dollars in savings for every dollar paid to a consultant pharmacist, as well as immeasurable gains in the quality-of-life column.

What's more, the total savings would go far, far beyond the savings in drug costs. Many of the patients I see in nursing homes and in hospice after admission return home after their drug therapy is reviewed and adjusted appropriately.

Medicare Part A patients who come into the nursing home from a hospital typically arrive with drug regimens that are hard to believe. Some of the patients I see come from the hospital with seventeen or eighteen different medications on board, a situation that invariably is at the root of serious — and often life-threatening — medical problems. These patients, many of them eighty-five years of age or older, need immediate help in the form of a drug therapy regimen that will help them get well — or at least better. Such a heavy medication load is a true indicator that the hospital's pharmacist pretty much wields a rubber stamp, doing little or nothing in the way of oversight. On average, independent consultant pharmacists like me will reduce the seventeen or eighteen medications to something in the neighborhood of four to six, stop all the adverse events going on, and allow the patient to recover from the drug-induced problems and respond more favorably to the overall treatment. You rarely if ever see this done by consultant pharmacists with corporate overlords.

The erosion of quality clinical-pharmacy services by independently owned nursing homes — which were bought up by the big corporate nursing home chains — was a large part of the reason behind my decision in 2000 to sell my consultant firm. Since then, I've continued to work as a consultant pharmacist for a manageable number of nursing homes that are independently owned or county-owned nursing home/hospital combinations. As I hope you've gathered by now, I'm challenged by the work and enjoy coming to know the people I help. The three nursing homes on my "circuit" these days have about four hundred patients, and each month I write up drug therapy suggestions for these patients that go to about a dozen doctors.

In 2010 I wrote suggestions in those three facilities to stop drugs that, if followed, would have saved a total of $503,604. Administering fewer medications to patients also saves a lot of nurses' time — in this case, something like 1,779 hours' worth, which would represent an additional savings of at least $17,790. Then there's the fact that, on average, 65 percent of the drugs stopped are one-time orders and the remaining 35 percent are used month after month after month (sometimes until the patient dies). This brings the total savings in drug costs to nearly $2.3 million a year, and the total savings in labor costs to slightly more than $24,000 a year.

This works out to about $5,665 in savings per year, per resident, not even including the savings in labor costs. And that's just me: one consultant pharmacist working in just three nursing homes in Georgia.

There are sixteen thousand or so nursing homes in the United States, with a total of about 1.5 million residents. If you use my savings-per-resident-per-year figure of $5,665 as a rough proxy for what might be achieved nationwide, you end up with something like $8.5 billion a year. And that's only for the people who are in the nation's nursing homes.

At last count, there were 39.6 million people sixty-five years of age and older in the United States. Nearly all of them, my experience tells me, are candidates for the type of drug therapy reviews you've read about in this book. If these Americans could access the services of independent consultant pharmacists — those with no ties of any kind to pharmacy providers, nursing homes, nursing home pharmacies, or hospital pharmacies — who would be reimbursed directly by Medicare, Medicaid, or private insurers, the savings to the health care system would be unbelievable.

One major change has to occur to make this happen: Congress will have to vote to include pharmacists in the Social Security Act as health professionals. They aren't included now because the AMA and other physicians groups have fought to keep them out. As a doctor once put it to me, "We don't need to divide the pie up any more than it is."

Once this change is made and pharmacists are recognized as "health professionals," then consultant pharmacists can be paid directly through Medicare Part B, just as doctors are.

Although consultant pharmacists have been around for nearly fifty years now, they are, in my judgment, vastly underutilized because the suggestions they make can be so easily and cavalierly ignored by prescribing physicians. Through their professional associations, physicians argue that consultant pharmacists interfere with the practice of medicine, and some go so far as to accuse consultant pharmacists of being engaged in the practice of medicine. Both of these arguments are spurious, as there's not a single pharmacist in the United States who can write a prescription (unless he or she also happens to be a physician).

As I see it, the practice of medicine and the practice of pharmacy will have to embrace change if we are to continue providing the best possible care for our patients. And if we don't embrace change, a broken system will force the wrong kind of change on all of us.

EPILOGUE:
MISS LILLIAN

A few years ago, I was deeply honored when the American Society of Consultant Pharmacists (ASCP) decided to add my name to its lifetime achievement award. I've been deeply involved with this professional association from the very beginning and was a charter member at the time of its founding in 1969. That was just four years after the Social Security Amendments of 1965 created Medicare and set the stage for major changes in the way we care for older people. The new law required nursing homes that participate in the Medicare program to be able to access the services of a consultant pharmacist.

The Armon Neel Senior Care Pharmacist Award is designed to recognize individuals who, as the ASCP puts it, "apply their knowledge of geriatric pharmacotherapy on a daily basis through the practice of senior care pharmacy and thereby significantly improve the quality of life of the senior population."

When I went before my ASCP peers in 2009 to accept the first version of this newly renamed annual award, I decided to tell a story that illustrates how the work that pharmacists do, day in and day out, really can touch — and even save — lives.

Back in 2002, I was traveling to a little town in north Georgia, to a nursing home that I had been going to for almost twenty years. I had developed quite a friendship with many of the patients there as well as with many members of the facility's staff. Some of the patients had been there for quite a while because they just couldn't take care of themselves at home.

It happened to be Valentine's Day. I've always made it a habit to stop by the CVS and buy all the stuff they have on sale for Valentine's Day so that I can take it to the nursing home and give something to all the patients.

As I went into the nursing home, one of the nurses called me aside and said, "One of your friends is dying."

"Who?" I asked.

"Miss Lillian's dying," she said. "She's had a stroke, and all the family's been called in." Now, this was quite a blow, as I had grown fond of this sweet little eighty-six-year-old lady named Lillian. Whenever I came to the nursing home, she'd always have a surprise for me.

As it happened, I'd bought a box of heart-shaped chocolates for Miss Lillian at the CVS. I took them down to her room, where she was lying in the bed unconscious. Her family was all around, and I leaned over and kissed her on the forehead. And I said, "I've brought you this box of Whitman's chocolates, and if you're not sitting on the side of the bed when I leave this afternoon, I'm going to take it home with me."

I turned around and walked back down to the nurses' station. I pulled her chart, and when I looked at it I saw, lo and behold, that about two weeks ago, the physician had just *stopped* the 10 milligrams of prednisone that she'd been taking every day for years and years. So I told the nurse, "I don't believe she's had a stroke; I believe she's in HPA." (That's the acronym for hypothalamic-pituitary-adrenal suppression, a condition that can lead to the total shut-down of the body's organ systems.)

And so the nurse went down and told the daughter, who came back up to see me. Just after she got there, the physician happened to arrive. When I explained what I thought was going on, the doctor made it clear that he wasn't really pleased with my intervention. "What have you got to lose?" I asked. "I think if we just put some cortisone in her IV fluids, we'll have her sitting on the side of the bed this afternoon."

At four o'clock that afternoon, as I was getting ready to leave, Miss Lillian's daughter came down and said, "Can you come back to the room for a minute?" And so I walked back to the room, and there I saw Miss Lillian sitting on the side of the bed.

Miss Lillian looked at me and winked, and I winked back at her. As I left the room, her daughter came up and thanked me, saying, "You're doing God's work." I got in my car, and all the way back home I was thinking about what I've heard all my career, that I'm doing God's work, and I couldn't really put my finger on whether I was or not.

Well, when Saint Patrick's Day came around, I went back to the nursing home. I stopped by the CVS, of course, to get a funny hat and all the green candy and stuff to hand out in the nursing home. As I walked in, there came Miss Lillian down the hall with a six-pack of Diet Dr Pepper and a jar of peanuts — two of my favorite things.

As I went to work in the nurses' station,

she came and sat down beside me. "You know what?" she said. "My husband died in 1957. You're the first man to give me a box of Valentine's Day candy since he died, and I love you for it. You saved my life."

"No, Miss Lillian," I said. "I didn't save your life. I just happened to be the messenger that brought the good news."

"Well," she said, "you saved my life, and I can't ever thank you enough for that." She was holding my hand, and as I looked at her, I could see tears rolling down her face. And I suddenly realized what she and tens of thousands before her had done: they'd opened up the doors of their hearts and allowed me to reach in and touch their souls.

And then I thought, "Well, maybe, just maybe, I really am doing God's work."

TAKING STOCK:
A SELF-ASSESSMENT QUIZ

Please take a few moments to answer all nine questions in part 1 of this Self-Assessment Quiz, circling *Y* for yes or *N* for no. It's very important that you answer these questions as accurately as you can.

Next, review all of the medications listed in part 2 of this form, noting whether you are currently taking any of them by circling *Y* or *N,* as applicable. (Where appropriate, one or more brand names are included, as you may better recognize the drugs you are taking that way.)

If you're sixty-five years or older and find that you have circled *Y* for more than four of the items on the self-assessment, I'd recommend that you consult with a board-certified geriatric pharmacist. (To find one, see page 411.)

Medication-related problems can rob older people of their good health and quality of life just at the time they should be enjoying life the most. Working with your physician, a senior care pharmacist can help make sure that you're taking the right medications in the right doses — and at the same time dramatically reduce the risks of medication-related problems.

What better time to start than right now?

PART 1: PLEASE ANSWER EACH OF THESE QUESTIONS

1. ARE YOU CURRENTLY TAKING FIVE OR MORE MEDICATIONS? . . . **Y or N** . . . .

2. ARE YOU TAKING TWELVE OR MORE DOSES OF MEDICATIONS PER DAY? . . . **Y or N** . . . . . .

3. DO YOU TAKE MEDICATIONS FOR THREE OR MORE MEDICAL PROBLEMS? . . . **Y or N** . . . . .

4. HAVE YOUR MEDICATIONS — OR THE INSTRUCTIONS FOR TAKING THEM — CHANGED FOUR OR MORE TIMES THIS PAST YEAR? . . . **Y or N** . . . .

5. DOES MORE THAN ONE PHYSICIAN PRESCRIBE MEDICATIONS FOR YOU ON A REGULAR BASIS? . . . **Y or N** . . .

6. ARE YOUR PRESCRIPTIONS FILLED BY MORE THAN ONE PHARMACY? . . . **Y or N** . . . . .

7. DOES SOMEONE ELSE BRING YOUR MEDICATIONS TO YOUR HOME (SPOUSE, FRIEND, NEIGHBOR, DELIVERY PERSON, AND SO ON)? . . . **Y or N** . . . .

8. DO YOU FIND IT DIFFICULT TO FOLLOW YOUR MEDICATION REGIMEN, OR SOMETIMES DO YOU CHOOSE NOT TO? . . . **Y or N**. . . . .

9. ARE YOU TAKING ANY MEDICATION(S) WITHOUT KNOWING EXACTLY WHY IT'S BEEN PRESCRIBED FOR YOU? . . . **Y or N**. . . . .

PART 2: DO YOU TAKE ANY OF THESE MEDICATIONS?

CARBAMAZEPINE (TEGRETOL) . . .
   Y or N . . . .
LITHIUM (ESKALITH) . . . **Y or N** . .
PHENYTOIN (DILANTIN,
   PHENYTEK) . . . **Y or N** . . . . .
QUINIDINE (QUINIDEX) . . . **Y or N** .
WARFARIN (COUMADIN) . . . **Y or N** .
DIGOXIN (LANOXIN,
   LANOXICAPS) . . . **Y or N** . . . .
PHENOBARBITAL (SOLFOTON) . . .
   Y or N . . . .
PROCAINAMIDE (PROCANBID,
   PRONESTYL) . . . **Y or N** . . . . .
THEOPHYLLINE (THEO-DUR,
   THEO-24, SLO-BID, UNIPHYL) . . .
   Y or N . . . .
ALPHA-BLOCKERS (CARDURA,
   CATAPRES, HYTRIN, FLOMAX) . . .
   Y or N . . . .
LEVOTHYROXINE (SYNTHROID) . . .
   Y or N . . . .

BISPHOSPHONATES (BONIVA,
FOSAMAX, RECLAST) . . . **Y or N** .
STATIN DRUGS (LIPITOR, ZOCOR,
PRAVACHOL) . . . **Y or N**. . . . .
METFORMIN (GLUCOPHAGE) . . .
Y or N. . . . .
GLIPIZIDE (GLUCOTROL),
GLIMEPIRIDE (AMARYL),
GLYBURIDE (DIABETA) . . .
Y or N. . . . .
HYDROCHLOROTHIAZIDE (ESIDRIX,
HYDRODIURIL, MICROZIDE) . . .
Y or N. . . . .
NITROFURANTOIN
(MACRODANTIN) . . . **Y or N** . . .
NSAIDS (ADVIL, ALEVE, MOTRIN) . . .
Y or N. . . . .
ANTIHISTAMINES (BENADRYL,
ANTIVERT, TYLENOL PM,
SLEEP-EZE, DRAMAMINE) . . .
Y or N. . . . .
CIMETIDINE (TAGAMET) . . .
Y or N. . . . .
KETOCONAZOLE (ALL ORAL
ANTIFUNGAL DRUGS) . . . **Y or N** .

RESOURCES, READINGS, AND REFERENCES

How to Find a Consultant Pharmacist

A consultant pharmacist can be an important part of your health care team by helping you identify and resolve medication-related problems. If you're sixty or older, or trying to help a parent or other loved one in that age group, I recommend that you find a board-certified geriatric pharmacist who works with individual patients. Keep in mind, however, that many consultant pharmacists are employed by universities, hospitals, and other institutions and thus do not work with individuals.

The Commission for Certification in Geriatric Pharmacy (www.ccgp.org), which was created by the American Society of Consultant Pharmacists in 1997 to oversee its certification program, offers a state-by-state lookup tool (www.ccgp.org/consumer/locate.htm) to help you find such a pharmacist near you.

AARP's Ask the Pharmacist Column

As AARP's Ask the Pharmacist columnist, I regularly write about medication-related topics in a question-and-answer format. The questions come from visitors to the AARP Web site.

Here's just a sampling:

"Can the estrogen I apply to my skin spread to my baby granddaughter?"
"Do drugs for early-stage Alzheimer's work?"
"Can a drug for urinary tract infections build up to toxic levels in my body?"
"Are my mother's medications making her fall?"

You can read my answers at www.aarp.org/askthepharmacist. And while you're there, you can even ask a question of your own.

Worst Pills, Best Pills

WorstPills.org is a project of Public Citizen's Health Research Group, which has been directed by Sidney Wolfe, MD, since its creation in 1971.

Wolfe and his colleagues promote evidence-based, systemwide changes in health care policy, with a primary focus on banning or relabeling unsafe or ineffective drugs as well as encouraging greater transparency and accountability in the drug-approval process. As an independent, non-profit watchdog, Public Citizen does not accept funding from corporations, professional associations, or government agencies.

I've subscribed to the low-cost *Worst Pills, Best Pills* newsletter for as long as I can remember. The doctors and pharmacists who write for it expertly analyze the Food and Drug Administration's own data and provide independent and invaluable second opinions on issues of drug safety and efficacy.

The NNT

The statistic we call "number needed to treat," or NNT, aims to measure the effectiveness of a medication or other intervention by estimating how many patients need to be treated to have the desired therapeutic effect on one person.

A physician-created Web site (www.thennt .com) gathers a lot of NNTs in one place. They're assembled in more than twenty different categories, from cardiology to urology. In the latter category, for example, you can quickly learn that the prostate-specific antigen (PSA) test that's used to screen for prostate cancer does not help to prevent death from any cause — including prostate cancer — and harms one in five patients by generating false-positive results that lead to unnecessary prostate biopsies.

SUGGESTED READING

Abramson, MD, John. *Overdosed America: The Broken Promise of American Medicine.* New York: HarperCollins, 2004.

Angell, MD, Marcia. *The Truth About the Drug Companies: How They Deceive Us and What to Do About It.* New York: Random House, 2004.

Avorn, MD, Jerry. *Powerful Medicines: The Benefits, Risks, and Costs of Prescription Drugs.* New York: Knopf, 2004.

Brownlee, Shannon. *Overtreated: Why Too Much Medicine Is Making Us Sicker and Poorer.* New York: Bloomsbury, 2007.

Hadler, MD, Nortin M. *The Last Well Person: How to Stay Well Despite the Health-Care System.* Montreal and Kingston, Canada: McGill-Queen's University Press, 2004.

———. *Worried Sick: A Prescription for Health in an Overtreated America.* Chapel Hill, North Carolina: University of North Carolina Press, 2008.

Moynihan, Ray, and Alan Cassels. *Selling Sickness: How the World's Biggest Pharmaceutical Companies Are Turning Us All into*

Patients. New York: Nation Books, 2005.

Petersen, Melody. *Our Daily Meds: How the Pharmaceutical Companies Transformed Themselves into Slick Marketing Machines and Hooked the Nation on Prescription Drugs.* New York: Farrar, Straus and Giroux, 2008.

Wolfe, MD, Sidney M., Larry D. Sasich, PharmD, MPH, Peter Lurie, MD, MPH, et al. *Worst Pills, Best Pills: A Consumer's Guide to Avoiding Drug-Induced Death or Illness.* New York: Pocket Books, 2005.

Welch, MD, H. Gilbert, Lisa M. Schwartz, MD, and Steven Woloshin, MD. *Overdiagnosed: Making People Sick in the Pursuit of Health.* Boston: Beacon Press, 2011.

Woloshin, MD, MS, Steven, Lisa M. Schwartz, MD, MS, and H. Gilbert Welch, MD, MPH. *Know Your Chances: Understanding Health Statistics.* Berkeley, CA, and Los Angeles: University of California Press, 2008.

REFERENCES

Prologue: The Pharmacist Who Says No to Drugs

J. Lyle Bootman, Donald L. Harrison, and Emily Cox. "The Health Care Cost of Drug-Related Morbidity and Mortality in

Nursing Facilities." *Archives of Internal Medicine* 157:2089–2096, 1997.

Good-bye and Good Luck: Helping Yourself to Better Health

Jason Lazarou, Bruce H. Pomeranz, MD, and Paul N. Corey. "Incidence of Adverse Drug Reactions in Hospitalized Patients: A Meta-Analysis of Prospective Studies," *Journal of the American Medical Association* 279(15):1200–1205, 1998.

"More Doctors on the Care Team Correlates With Higher Risk of Adverse Drug Events in Seniors," Medco Health Solutions, Inc., September 13, 2006 (news release).

The State of Aging and Health in America 2004. Centers for Disease Control and Prevention and Merck Institute of Aging & Health, 2004.

Daniel S. Budnitz, MD, Nadine Shehab, Scott R. Kegler, and Chesley L. Richards, MD, "Medication Use Leading to Emergency Department Visits for Adverse Drug Events in Older Adults," *Annals of Internal Medicine* 147(11):755–765, 2007.

Things Change: Our Aging Bodies

Andrew S. Levey, MD, Juan P. Bosch, MD, Julia Breyer Lewis, MD, et al., "A More

Accurate Method To Estimate Glomerular Filtration Rate from Serum Creatinine: A New Prediction Equation," *Annals of Internal Medicine* 130(6):461–470, 1999.

Donald W. Cockcroft, MD, and Henry Gault, MD, "Prediction of Creatinine Clearance from Serum Creatinine," *Nephron* 16(1):31–41, 1976.

Gordon G. Liu and Dale B. Christensen, "The Continuing Challenge of Inappropriate Prescribing in the Elderly: An Update of the Evidence," *Journal of the American Pharmaceutical Association* 42(6):847–857, 2002.

Piling On: The Perils of Polypharmacy

Jane E. Brody, "The 'Poisonous Cocktail' of Multiple Drugs," *The New York Times,* September 18, 2007.

Roger J. Cadieux, MD, "Drug Interactions in the Elderly: How Multiple Drug Use Increases Risk Exponentially," *Journal of Postgraduate Medicine* 86(8):179–86, 1989.

Robyn M. Tamblyn, Peter J. McLeod, MD, Michal Abrahamowicz, and Réjean Laprise, "Do Too Many Cooks Spoil the Broth? Multiple Physician Involvement in Medical Management of Elderly Patients and Potentially Inappropriate Drug Com-

417

binations," *Canadian Medical Association Journal* 154(8):1177–1184, 1996.

Amit A. Shah, "Drugs You Might Stop: A Practical Approach to Medication Debridement," *Family Practice Decertification* 29(6):45, June 2007.

Sean D. Sullivan, David H. Kreling, and Thomas K. Hazlet, "Noncompliance with Medication Regimens and Subsequent Hospitalization: A Literature Analysis and Cost of Hospitalization Estimate," *Journal of Research in Pharmaceutical Economics* 2(2):19–33, 1990.

Doron Garfinkel, MD, and Derelie Mangin, "Feasibility Study of a Systematic Approach for Discontinuation of Multiple Medications in Older Adults: Addressing Polypharmacy," *Archives of Internal Medicine* 170(18):1648–1654, 2010.

Off-Limits for Older People: The Beers Criteria

Anne Harding, "Obituary: Mark H. Beers," *The Lancet* 373(9674):1518, 2009.

Mark H. Beers, MD, Joseph G. Ouslander, MD, Irving Rollingher, MD, David B. Reuben, MD, Jacqueline Brooks, and John C. Beck, MD, "Explicit Criteria for Determining Inappropriate Medication Use in Nursing Home Residents," *Archives of*

Internal Medicine 151(9):1825–1832, 1991.

Mark H. Beers, MD, "Explicit Criteria for Determining Potentially Inappropriate Medication Use by the Elderly: An Update," *Archives of Internal Medicine* 157(14):1531–1536, 1997.

Elizabeth Cohen, "Is Grandma Drugged Up?" CNN.com, May 28, 2008.

Karen M. Stockl, Lisa Le, Shaoang Zhang, and Ann S. M. Harada, "Clinical and Economic Outcomes Associated With Potentially Inappropriate Prescribing in the Elderly," *The American Journal of Managed Care* 16(1):e1–e10, 2010.

U.S. Department of Health and Human Services, Centers for Medicare and Medicaid Services, "Requirements for Long-Term Care Facilities," 42 *Code of Federal Regulations* §483.25, 2009.

Donna M. Fick, James W. Cooper, William E. Wade, Jennifer L. Waller, J. Ross Maclean, MD, and Mark H. Beers, MD, "Updating the Beers Criteria for Potentially Inappropriate Medication Use in Older Adults: Results of a U.S. Consensus Panel of Experts," *Archives of Internal Medicine* 163(22):2716–2724, 2003.

Mark Beers, MD, Jerry Avorn, MD, Stephen B. Soumerai, Daniel E. Everitt, MD,

David S. Sherman, and Susanne Salem, "Psychoactive Medication Use in Intermediate-Care Facility Residents," *Journal of the American Medical Association* 260(20):3016–3020, 1988.

G. Caleb Alexander, MD, Sarah A. Gallagher, Anthony Mascola, Rachael M. Moloney, Randall S. Stafford, "Increasing Off-Label Use of Antipsychotic Medications in the United States, 1995–2008," *Pharmacoepidemiology and Drug Safety* 20(2):177–184, 2011.

Jerry H. Gurwitz, MD, Terry S. Field, Jerry Avorn, MD, Danny McCormick, MD, et al., "Incidence and Preventability of Adverse Drug Events in the Nursing Home Setting," *American Journal of Medicine* 109(2):87–94, 2000.

Jerry H. Gurwitz, MD, Terry S. Field, James Judge, MD, Paula Rochon, MD, et al., "The Incidence of Adverse Drug Effects in Two Large Academic Long-Term Care Facilities," *American Journal of Medicine* 118(3):251–258, 2005.

Wayne A. Ray, Marie R. Griffin, MD, William Schaffner, MD, David K. Baugh, L. Joseph Melton, MD, "Psychotropic Drug Use and the Risk of Hip Fracture," *New England Journal of Medicine* 316:363–369, 1987.

Purushottam B. Thapa, Kelly G. Brockman, Patricia Gideon, Randy L. Fought, and Wayne A. Ray, "Injurious Falls in Nonambulatory Nursing Home Residents: A Comparative Study of Circumstances, Incidence, and Risk Factors," *Journal of the American Geriatrics Society* 44(3):273–278, 1996.

U.S. Department of Health and Human Services, Office of Inspector General. *Medicare Atypical Antipsychotic Drug Claims for Elderly Nursing Home Residents,* May 2011.

Tracy Weber and Charles Ornstein, "Doctors Avoid Penalties in Suits Against Medical Firms," *ProPublica.org,* September 16, 2011; Tracy Weber and Charles Ornstein, "This Won't Hurt a Bit," *Washington Post,* September 18, 2011, p. G1.

John C. Woolcott, Kathryn J. Richardson, Matthew O. Wiens, Bhavini Patel, Judith Marin, Karim M. Khan, MD, and Carlo A. Marra, "Meta-Analysis of the Impact of Nine Medication Classes of Falls in Elderly Persons," *Archives of Internal Medicine* 169(21):1952–1960, 2009.

National Institutes of Health, National Heart, Lung, and Blood Institute, "NHLBI Stops Trial of Estrogen Plus Progestin Due to Increased Breast Cancer

Risk, Lack of Overall Health Benefit," July 9, 2002 [news release].

Loren Laine, MD, "GI Risk and Risk Factors of NSAIDs," *Journal of Cardiovascular Pharmacology* 47(S1):S60–S66, 2006.

Rashmi Shukla, Nigel I. Jowett, MD, D.R. Thompson, and J.E.F. Pohl, "Side Effects with Amiodarone Therapy," *Postgraduate Medical Journal* 70(825):492–498, 1994.

Antiplatelet Trialists' Collaboration, "Secondary Prevention of Vascular Disease by Prolonged Antiplatelet Treatment," *British Medical Journal* (Clinical Research Edition) 296(6618):320–331, 1988.

Troy L. Thompson, II, MD, Christopher M. Filley, MD, Wayne D. Mitchell, Kathleen M. Culig, Mary LoVerde, and Richard L. Byyny, MD, "Lack of Efficacy of Hydergine in Patients with Alzheimer's Disease," *New England Journal of Medicine* 323:445–448, 1990.

Eric B. Larsen, MD, "Geriatric Medicine," *Journal of the American Medical Association* 265(23):3125–3126, 1991.

Carol Coupland, Paula Dhiman, Richard Morriss, Antony Arthur, Garry Barton, Julia Hippisley-Cox, "Antidepressant Use and Risk of Adverse Outcomes in Older People: Population-Based Cohort Study,"

British Medical Journal 343:bmj.d4551, 2011.

Marco Pahor, MD, Jack M. Guralnik, MD, Maria-Chiara Corti, MD, Daniel J. Foley, Pierugo Carbonin, MD, and Richard J. Havlik, MD, "Long-Term Survival and Use of Antihypertensive Medications in Older Persons," *Journal of the American Geriatrics Society* 43(11):1191–1197, 1995.

Jean-Pierre Desager, "Clinical Pharmacokinetics of Ticlopidine," *Clinical Pharmacokinetics* 26:347–355, 1994.

Off the Charts: Do You Really Need Those Blood-Pressure Drugs?

Randy Wexler, MD, Christopher Taylor, Adam Pleister, MD, and David Feldman, MD, "When Your Patient's Blood Pressure Won't Come Down," *Journal of Family Practice* 58(12):640–645, 2009.

Lars Osterberg, MD, and Terrence Blaschke, MD, "Adherence to Medication," *New England Journal of Medicine* 353:487–497, 2005.

Bimal V. Patel, Rosemay A. Remigio-Baker, Devi Mehta, Patrick Thiebaud, Feride Frech-Tamas, and Ronald Preblick, "Effects of Initial Antihypertensive Drug Class on Patient Persistence and Compliance in a Usual-Care Setting in the United States," *Journal of Clinical Hypertension* 9(9):692–700, 2007.

Peter V. Dicpinigaitis, MD, "Angiotensin-Converting Enzyme Inhibitor-Induced Cough: ACCP [American College of Chest Physicians] Evidence-Based Clinical Practice Guidelines," *Chest* 129(1 supplement):169S–173S, 2006.

Balraj S. Heran, Michelle MY Wong, Inderjit K. Heran, and James M. Wright, MD, "Blood Pressure Lowering Efficacy of Angiotensin Receptor Blockers for Primary Hypertension," Cochrane Database of Systematic Reviews, 2008.

James M. Mason, Heather O. Dickinson, Donald J. Nicolson, Fiona Campbell, Gary A. Ford, and Bryan Williams, "The Diabetogenic Potential of Thiazide-Type Diuretic and Beta-Blocker Combinations in Patients with Hypertension," *Journal of Hypertension* 23(10):1777–1781, 2005.

Finlay A. McAlister, MD, Jianguo Zhang, Marcello Tonelli, MD, Scott Klarenbach, MD, Braden J. Manns, MD, and Brenda R. Hemmelgarn, MD, "The Safety of Combining Angiotensin-Converting-Enzyme Inhibitors with Angiotensin-Receptor Blockers in Elderly Patients: A Population-Based Longitudinal Analysis,"

Journal of the Canadian Medical Association 183(6):655–662, 2011.

José Agustin Arguedas, MD, Marco I. Perez, MD, and James M. Wright, MD, "Treatment Blood Pressure Targets for Hypertension," Cochrane Database of Systematic Reviews, 2009.

Lennart Hansson, MD, Alberto Zanchetti, MD, S. George Carruthers, MD, Björn Dahlöf, MD, et al., "Effects of Intensive Blood-Pressure Lowering and Low-Dose Aspirin in Patients With Hypertension: Principal Results of the Hypertension Optimal Treatment (HOT) Randomised Trial," *Lancet* 351:1755–1762, 1998.

Frank M. Sacks, MD, Laura P. Svetkey, MD, William M. Vollmer, Lawrence J. Appel, MD, et al., "Effects on Blood Pressure of Reduced Dietary Sodium and the Dietary Approaches to Stop Hypertension (DASH) Diet," *New England Journal of Medicine* 344:3–10, 2001.

Seamus Whelton, Amanda D. Hyre, Bonnie Pedersen, Yeonjoo Yi, Paul K. Whelton, and Jiang He, "Effect of Dietary Fiber Intake on Blood Pressure: A Meta-Analysis of Randomized, Controlled Clinical Trials," *American Journal of Hypertension* 23(3):475–481, 2005.

Phantom Killers: NSAIDS (Nonsteroidal Anti-Inflammatory Drugs)

Gurkirpal Singh, MD, "Recent Considerations in Nonsteroidal Anti-Inflammatory Drug Gastrophy," *American Journal of Medicine* 105(1B):31S–38S, 2008.

M. Michael Wolfe, MD, David R. Lichtenstein, MD, and Gurkirpal Singh, MD, "Gastrointestinal Toxicity of Nonsteroidal Antiinflammatory Drugs," *New England Journal of Medicine* 340:1888–1899, 1999.

Loren A. Laine, MD, "The Gastrointestinal Effects of Nonselective NSAIDs and COX-2-Selective Inhibitors," *Seminars in Arthritis and Rheumatism* 32:25–32, 2002.

Leif E. Dahlberg, Ingar Holme, Kjetil Høye, and Bo Ringertz, "A Randomized, Multicentre, Double-Blind, Parallel-Group Study to Assess the Adverse Event-Related Discontinuation Rate with Celecoxib and Diclofenac in Elderly Patients with Osteoarthritis," *Scandinavian Journal of Rheumatology* 38(2):133–143, 2009.

Shuji Asada, Yasuhiro Okumura, Akio Matsumoto, Ichiro Hirata, and Saburo Ohshiba, "Correlation of Gastric Mucous Volume With Levels of Five Prostaglandins After Gastric Mucosal Injuries by NSAIDs," *Journal of Clinical Gastroenterol-*

ogy 12(1):S125–S130, 1990.

David Y. Graham, MD, Antone R. Opekun, Field F. Willingham, MD, and Wagar A. Qureshi, MD, "Visible Small-Intestine Mucosal Injury in Chronic NSAID Users," *Clinical Gastroenterology and Hepatology,* 3(1):55–59, 2005.

Sven Trelle, MD, Stephan Reichenbach, MD, Simon Wandel, Pius Hildebrand, MD, Beatrice Tschannen, Peter M. Villiger, Matthias Egger, and Peter Jüni, "Cardiovascular Safety of Non-Steroidal Anti-Inflammatory Drugs: Network Meta-Analysis," *BMJ* 342:bmj.c7086, 2011.

John P. Forman, MD, Eric B. Rimm, and Gary C. Curhan, MD, "Frequency of Analgesic Use and Risk of Hypertension Among Men," *Archives of Internal Medicine* 167(4):394–399, 2007.

William B. White, MD, "Cardiovascular Effects of the Cyclooxygenase Inhibitors," *Hypertension* 49(3):408–418, 2007.

Patrick R. Pfau, MD, and Gary R. Lichtenstein, MD, "NSAIDs and Alcohol: Never the Twain Shall Mix?" *American Journal of Gastroenterology* 94:3098–3101, 1999.

American College of Gastroenterology, *Understanding Ulcers, NSAIDs, and GI Bleeding: A Consumer Health Guide.*

Ronald I. Shorr, MD, Wayne A. Ray, James

R. Daugherty, and Marie R. Griffin, MD, "Concurrent Use of Nonsteroidal Anti-Inflammatory Drugs and Oral Anticoagulants Places Elderly Persons at High Risk for Hemorrhagic Peptic Ulcer Disease," *Archives of Internal Medicine* 153(14):1665–1670, 1993.

Meredith B. Rosenthal, Ernst R. Berndt, Julie M. Donohue, Richard G. Frank, and Arnold M. Epstein, MD, "Promotion of Prescription Drugs to Consumers," *New England Journal of Medicine* 346(7):498–505, 2002.

Carolanne Dai, Randall S. Stafford, MD, and G. Caleb Alexander, M.D, "National Trends in Cyclooxygenase-2 Inhibitor Use Since Market Release: Nonselective Diffusion of a Selectively Cost-Effective Innovation," *Archives of Internal Medicine* 165:171–177, 2005.

Proton Pump Inhibitors: The Miracle Drugs That Aren't

Nimish Vakil, MD, Sander V. van Zanten, MD, Peter Kahrilas, MD, John Dent, MD, and Roger Jones, MD, "The Montreal Definition and Classification of Gastro-Esophageal Reflux Disease: A Global Evidence-Based Consensus," *American Journal of Gastroenterology* 101(8):1900–

1920, 2006.

Christina Reimer, MD, and Peter Bytzer, MD, "Clinical Trial: Long-Term Use of Proton Pump Inhibitors in Primary-Care Patients — A Cross-Sectional Analysis of 901 Patients," *Alimentary Pharmacology & Therapeutics* 30(7):725–732, 2009.

John Dent, MD, Hashem B. El-Serag, MD, Mari-Ann Wallander, and Saga Johansson, "Epidemiology of Gastrooesophageal Reflux Disease: A Systematic Review," *Gut* 54(5):710–717, 2005.

Eva M. van Soest, Peter D. Siersema, MD, Jeanne P. Dieleman, Miriam C.J.M. Sturkenboom, MD, and Ernst J. Kuipers, "Persistence and Adherence to Proton Pump Inhibitors in Daily Clinical Practice," *Alimentary Pharmacology & Therapeutics* 24(2):377–385, 2006.

Ernst J. Kuipers, MD, "Proton Pump Inhibitors and Gastric Neoplasia," *Gut* 55(9):1217–1221, 2006.

Christina Reimer, MD, Bo Søndergaard, MD, Linda Hilsted, MD, and Peter Bytzer, MD, "Proton-Pump Inhibitor Therapy Induces Acid-Related Symptoms in Healthy Volunteers After Withdrawal of Therapy," *Gastroenterology* 137(1):80–87, 2009.

Ronnie Fass, MD, and Daniel Sifrim, MD,

"Management of Heartburn Not Responding to Proton Pump Inhibitors," *Gut* 58(2):295–309, 2009.

Folke Johnsson, MD, Jan G. Hatlebakk, MD, Ann-Charlotte Klintenberg, and Jonas Róman, "Symptom-Relieving Effect of Esomeprazole 40 mg Daily in Patients With Heartburn," *Scandinavian Journal of Gastroenterology* 38(4):347–353, 2003.

Caroline Helwick, "Study Supports Link Between PPI Use and Hip Fracture," *GI & Hepatology News,* September 2011, p. 4.

Katie S. Nason, MD, Promporn Paula Wichienkuer, MD, Omar Awais, MD, Matthew J. Schuchert, MD, et al., "Gastroesophageal Reflux Disease Symptom Severity, Proton Pump Inhibitor Use, and Esophageal Carcinogenesis," *Archives of Surgery* 146(7):851–858, 2011.

Sandra Dial, MD, J.A. Chris Delaney, Verena Schneider, and Samy Suissa, "Proton Pump Inhibitor Use and Risk of Community-Acquired Clostridium Difficile-Associated Disease Defined by Prescription for Oral Vancomycin Therapy," *Canadian Medical Association Journal* 175(7):745–748, 2006.

Amy Linsky, MD, Kalpana Gupta, MD, Elizabeth V. Lawler, Jennifer R. Fonda, and John A. Hermos, MD, "Proton Pump Inhibitors and Risk for Recurrent *Clostridium difficile* Infection," *Archives of Internal Medicine* 170(9):772–778.

Michael D. Howell, MD, Victor Novack, MD, Philip Grgurich, Diane Soulliard, Lena Novack, Michael Pencina, and Daniel Talmor, MD, "Iatrogenic Gastric Acid Suppression and the Risk of Nosocomial *Clostridium difficile* Infection," *Archives of Internal Medicine* 170(9):784–790, 2010.

M.N. Choudhry, Handrean Soran, and Hisham M. Ziglam, MD, "Overuse and Inappropriate Prescribing of Proton Pump Inhibitors in Patients with *Clostridium Difficile*-Associated Disease," *QJM: An International Journal of Medicine* 101(6):445–448, 2008.

Farrah Ibrahim J. Al-Tureihi, MD, Ali Hassoun, MD, Gisele Wolf-Klein, MD, and Henry Isenberg, "Albumin, Length of Stay, and Proton Pump Inhibitors: Key Factors in *Clostridium Difficile*-Associated Disease in Nursing Home Patients," *Journal of the American Medical Directors Association* 6(2):105–108, 2005.

Robert J.F. Laheij, Miriam C.J.M. Sturkenboom, Robert-Jan Hassing, Jeanne Dieleman, Bruno H.C. Stricker, MD, and Jan

B.M.J. Jansen, MD, "Risk of Community-Acquired Pneumonia and Use of Gastric Acid-Suppressive Drugs," *Journal of the American Medical Association* 292(16): 1955–1960, 2004.

Sinem Ezgi Gulmez, MD, Anette Holm, MD, Henrik Frederiksen, MD, Thøger Gorm Jensen, MD, Court Pedersen, and Jesper Hallas, "Use of Proton Pump Inhibitors and the Risk of Community-Acquired Pneumonia: A Population-Based Case-Control Study," *Archives of Internal Medicine* 167(9):950–955, 2007.

Monika Sarkar, MD, Sean Hennessy, and Yu-Xiao Yang, MD, "Proton-Pump Inhibitor Use and the Risk for Community-Acquired Pneumonia," *Annals of Internal Medicine* 149(6):391–398, 2008.

Shoshana J. Herzig, MD, Michael D. Howell, MD, Long H. Ngo, and Edward R. Marcantonio, MD, "Acid-Suppressive Medication Use and the Risk for Hospital-Acquired Pneumonia," *Journal of the American Medical Association* 301(20): 2120–2128, 2009.

Kimberly A. Skarupski, Christine Tangney, Hong Li, Bichun Ouyang, Denis A. Evans, and Martha Clare Morris, "Longitudinal Association of Vitamin B-6, Folate, and

Vitamin B-12 with Depressive Symptoms Among Older Adults Over Time," *American Journal of Clinical Nutrition* 92(2):330–335, 2010.

John L. Wallace, MD, Stephanie Syer, Emmanuel Denou, Giada de Palma, et al., "Proton Pump Inhibitors Exacerbate NSAID-Induced Small Intestinal Injury by Inducing Dysbiosis," *Gastroenterology* 141(4):1312–1322.e5, 2011.

McMaster University, Faculty of Health Sciences, "McMaster Study Finds More Gut Reaction to Arthritis Drugs," September 2, 2011 (news release).

Shoshana J. Herzig, MD, Byron P. Vaughn, MD, Michael D. Howell, MD, Long H. Ngo, and Edward R. Marcantonio, MD, "Acid-Suppressive Medication Use and the Risk for Nosocomial Gastrointestinal Tract Bleeding," *Archives of Internal Medicine* 171(11):991–997, 2011.

Ricardo de Souza Pereira, "Regression of Gastroesophageal Reflux Disease Symptoms Using Dietary Supplementation with Melatonin, Vitamins, and Aminoacids: Comparison with Omeprazole," *Journal of Pineal Research* 41:195–200, 2006.

Kenneth E.L. McColl, MD, and Derek Gillen, MD, "Evidence That Proton-Pump Inhibitor Therapy Induces the

Symptoms It Is Used to Treat," *Gastroenterology* 137(1):20–39, 2009.

Statin Roulette: Drugs of Last Resort

U.S. Department of Health and Human Services, Centers for Disease Control and Prevention, National Center for Health Statistics. *Health, United States, 2010: With Special Feature on Death and Dying.* Hyattsville, Maryland: National Center for Health Statistics, 2011.

Michelle Roberts, "Statin-Fortified Drinking Water?" BBC News Online, August 1, 2004.

Robert Lemmon, MD, "Overrated Medications Series: No. 2 — Statins for Primary Prevention of Cardiovascular Diseases," *Bittersweet Medicine: Opinions from a Family Doctor,* www.bittersweetmedicine.com, March 26, 2010.

John Abramson, MD, and James Wright, MD, "Are Lipid-Lowering Guidelines Evidence-Based?" *Lancet* 369(9557):168–169, 2007

Fiona Taylor, MD, Kirsten Ward, Theresa H.M. Moore, Margaret Burke, George Davey Smith, Juan-Pablo Casas, MD, and Shah Ebrahim, MD, "Statins for the Primary Prevention of Cardiovascular Disease," Cochrane Database of Systematic Reviews, 2011.

Kausik K. Ray, MD, Sreenivasa Rao Konda-pally Seshasai, MD, Sebhat Erqou, MD, Peter Sever, et al., "Statins and All-Cause Mortality in High-Risk Primary Prevention: A Meta-analysis of 11 Randomized Controlled Trials Involving 65,229 Participants," *Archives of Internal Medicine* 170(12):1024–1031, 2010.

Lee A. Green, MD, "Cholesterol-Lowering Therapy for Primary Prevention: Still Much We Don't Know," *Archives of Internal Medicine,* 170(12):1007–1008, 2010.

Georgirene D. Vladutiu, Zachary Simmons, MD, Paul J. Isackson, Mark Tarnopolsky, MD, et al., "Genetic Risk Factors Associated With Lipid-Lowering Drug-Induced Myopathies," *Muscle & Nerve* 34(2):153–62, 2006.

Matthew F. Muldoon, MD, Christopher M. Ryan, Susan M. Sereika, Janine D. Flory, and Stephen B. Manuck, "Randomized Trial of the Effects of Simvastatin on Cognitive Functioning in Hypercholesterolemic Adults," *American Journal of Medicine* 117(11):823–829, 2004.

Matthew F. Muldoon, MD, Steven D. Barger, Christopher M. Ryan, Janine D. Flory, et al., "Effects of Lovastatin on Cognitive Function and Psychological

Well-Being," *American Journal of Medicine* 108(7):538–546, 2000.

Marcella B. Evans, Beatrice A. Golomb, MD, "Statin-Associated Adverse Cognitive Effects: Survey Results From 171 Patients," *Pharmacotherapy* 29(7):800–811, 2009.

Naveed Sattar, David Preiss, Heather M. Murray, Paul Welsh, et al., "Statins and Risk of Incident Diabetes: A Collaborative Meta-Analysis of Randomised Statin Trials," *The Lancet* 375(9716):735–742, 2010.

David Preiss, Sreenivasa Rao Kondapally Seshasai, MD, Paul Welsh, Sabina A. Murphy, et al., "Risk of Incident Diabetes with Intensive-Dose Compared with Moderate-Dose Statin Therapy," *Journal of the American Medical Association* 305(24):2556–2564, 2011.

M. Brandon Westover, MD, Matt T. Bianchi, MD, Mark H. Eckman, MD, and Steven M. Greenberg, MD, "Statin Use Following Intracerebral Hemorrhage: A Decision Analysis," *Archives of Neurology* 68(5):573–579, 2011.

Larry B. Goldstein, MD, "Statins After Intracerebral Hemorrhage: To Treat or Not to Treat," *Archives of Neurology* 68(5):561–562, 2011.

Kenneth E. Thummel and Grant R. Wilkinson, "In Vitro and In Vivo Drug Interactions Involving Human CYP3A," *Annual Review of Pharmacology and Toxicology* 38:389–430, 1998.

Yasuhiro Uno, Hideki Fujino, Go Kito, Tetsuya Kamataki, and Ryoichi Nagata, "CYP2C76, a Novel Cytochrome P450 in Cynomolgus Monkey, Is a Major CYP2C in Liver, Metabolizing Tolbutamide and Testosterone," *Molecular Pharmacology* 70(2):477–486, 2006.

Line Kirkeby Petersen, MD, Kaare Christensen, MD, and Jakob Kragstrup, MD, "Lipid-Lowering Treatment to the End? A Review of Observational Studies and RCTs on Cholesterol and Mortality in 80+-Year-Olds," *Age and Ageing* 39(6):674–680, 2010.

Beatrice A. Golomb, MD, John J. McGraw, Marcella A. Evans, and Joel E. Dimsdale, MD, "Physician Response to Patient Reports of Adverse Drug Effects: Implications for Patient-Targeted Adverse Effect Surveillance," *Drug Safety* 30(8)669–675, 2007.

Markus G. Mohaupt, MD, Richard H. Karas, MD, Eduard B. Babiychuk, Verónica Sanchez-Freire, et al., "Association Between Statin-Associated Myopathy and Skeletal Muscle Damage," *CMAJ* 181(1–2):E11–E18, 2009.

James Shepherd, MD, Stuart M. Cobbe, MD, Ian Ford, Christopher G. Isles, MD, et al., "Prevention of Coronary Heart Disease with Pravastatin in Men with Hypercholesterolemia," *New England Journal of Medicine* 333:1301–1308, 1995.

Fiona Taylor, MD, Kirsten Ward, Theresa H.M. Moore, Margaret Burke, George Davey Smith, Juan-Pablo Casas, MD, and Shah Ebrahim, MD, "Statins for the Primary Prevention of Cardiovascular Disease," Cochrane Database of Systematic Reviews, 2011.

Karin Ried, Peter Fakler, "Protective Effect of Lycopene on Serum Cholesterol and Blood Pressure: Meta-Analyses of Intervention Trials," *Maturitas* 68(4):299–310, 2011.

Down and Out: Drug-Induced Falls

Bruce H. Alexander, Frederick P. Rivara, MD, and Marsha E. Wolf, "The Cost and Frequency of Hospitalization for Fall-Related Injuries in Older Adults," *American Journal of Public Health* 82(7):1020–3, 1992.

Daniel A. Sterling, MD, Judith A. O'Connor, and John Bonadies, MD, "Geriatric

Falls: Injury Severity Is High and Disproportionate to Mechanism," *Journal of Trauma: Injury, Infection, and Critical Care* 2001;50(1):116–9.

Cynthia L. Leibson, Anna N.A. Toteson, Sherine E. Gabriel, MD, Jeanine E. Ransom, and L. Joseph Melton III, MD. "Mortality, Disability, and Nursing Home Use for Persons with and without Hip Fracture: A Population-Based Study," *Journal of the American Geriatrics Society* 50(10):1644–50, 2002.

Judy Steed, "Drugged-Out Seniors a Prescription for Disaster," *Toronto Star,* November 11, 2008, p. A1.

Ngaire Kerse, Leon Flicker, MD, Jon J. Pfaff, Brian Draper, MD, et al., "Falls, Depression and Antidepressants in Later Life: A Large Primary Care Appraisal," *PLoS ONE,* 3(6):e2423, 2008.

Yvonne L. Michael, Evelyn P. Whitlock, MD, Jennifer S. Lin, MD, Rongwei Fu, Elizabeth A. O'Connor, and Rachel Gold, "Primary Care–Relevant Interventions to Prevent Falling in Older Adults: A Systematic Evidence Review for the U.S. Preventive Services Task Force," *Annals of Internal Medicine* 153(12):815–825, 2010.

Janet A. Wilson, MD, and W.J. MacLennan, MD, "Review: Drug-Induced Parkinsonism in Elderly Patients," *Age and Ageing,* 18(3):208–210, 1989.

Yong Chen, MD, Becky A. Briesacher, Terry S. Field, Jennifer Tjia, MD, Denys T. Lau, and Jerry H. Gurwitz, MD, "Unexplained Variation Across U.S. Nursing Homes in Antipsychotic Prescribing Rates," *Archives of Internal Medicine* 170(1):89–95, 2010.

Sarah D. Berry, MD, Murray A. Mittleman, MD, Yuqing Zhang, Daniel H. Solomon, MD, Lewis A. Lipsitz, MD, and Douglas P. Kiel, MD, "Diuretics Increase Morbidity and Risk of Falls in the Elderly," *Reactions Weekly* (1356):5, 2011.

Evandro S.F. Coutinho, Astrid Fletcher, MD, Katia V. Bloch, and Laura C. Rodrigues, MD, "Risk Factors for Falls With Severe Fracture in Elderly People Living in a Middle-Income Country: A Case Control Study," *BMC Geriatrics* 8:21, 2008.

Judith Hegeman, Bart J.F. van den Bemt, Jacques Duysens, MD, and Jacques van Limbeek, MD, "NSAIDs and the Risk of Accidental Falls in the Elderly: A Systematic Review," *Drug Safety* 32(6):489–498, 2009.

Marije E. Müller, Nathalie van der Velde, MD, Jaap W.M. Krulder, MD, and Tischa J.M. van der Cammen, MD, "Syncope and Falls Due to Timolol Eye Drops," *BMJ* 332(7547):960–961, 2006

Roland Grad, MD, "More Evidence Linking Benzodiazepines and Falls," *Canadian Family Physician* 43:1367–1368, 1997.

The Bone-Scare Drugs: What You Should Know About Bisphosphonates

Nancy Dow, "Proactive Approach to Health," *The* [Portland] *Oregonian,* July 12, 2006, p. C1.

Margery Gass, MD, and Bess Dawson-Hughes, MD, "Preventing Osteoporosis-Related Fractures: An Overview," *American Journal of Medicine* 119(4 Suppl. 1):S3–S11, 2006.

Jane E. Brody, "Hailed and Feared Cortisone Now Safer and More Varied," *The New York Times,* January 21, 1981, p. C1.

Eric L. Matteson, MD, and Janis Larson Brown, MD, "A Patient Remembers the Miracle Drug Cortisone 50 Years Later," *Minnesota Medicine* 85(6):12–15, 2002.

Yu-Xiao Yang, MD, James D. Lewis, MD, Solomon Epstein, MD, and David C. Metz, MD, "Long-Term Proton Pump Inhibitor Therapy and Risk of Hip Fracture," *Journal of the American Medical Association* 296(24):2947–2953, 2006.

Diane K. Wysowski and Jennie T. Chang,

"Alendronate and Risedronate: Reports of Severe Bone, Joint, and Muscle Pain," *Archives of Internal Medicine* 165(3):346–347, 2005.

Jane Green, Gabriela Czanner, Gillian Reeves, Joanna Watson, Lesley Wise, and Valerie Beral, MD, "Oral Bisphosphonates and Risk of Cancer of Oesophagus, Stomach, and Colorectum: Case-Control Analysis within a U.K. Primary Care Cohort," *BMJ* 341:c4444, 2010.

Chris R. Cardwell, Christian C. Abnet, Marie M. Cantwell, and Liam J. Murray, MD, "Exposure to Oral Bisphosphonates and Risk of Esophageal Cancer," *Journal of the American Medical Association* 304(6):657–663, 2010.

Amir Qaseem, MD, Vincenza Snow, MD, Paul Shekelle, MD, Robert Hopkins, Jr., MD, Mary Ann Forciea, MD, and Douglas K. Owens, MD, "Pharmacologic Treatment of Low Bone Density or Osteoporosis to Prevent Fractures: A Clinical Practice Guideline from the American College of Physicians," *Annals of Internal Medicine* 149(6):404–415, 2008.

"Jury Says Merck Must Pay $8 Million in Fosamax Case," *New York Times,* June 26, 2010, p. B2.

Parish P. Sedghizadeh, Kyle Stanley, Matthew Caligiuri, Shawn Hofkes, Brad Lowry, and Charles F. Shuler, "Oral Bisphosphonate Use and the Prevalence of Osteonecrosis of the Jaw," *Journal of the American Dental Association* 140(1):61–66, 2009.

Salvatore L. Ruggiero, MD, and Bhoomi Mehrotra, MD, "Bisphosphonate-Related Osteonecrosis of the Jaw: Diagnosis, Prevention, and Management," *Annual Review of Medicine* 60:85–96, 2009.

Vandana Kumar, Barry Pass, Steven A. Guttenberg, MD, John Ludlow, Robert W. Emery, Donald A. Tyndall, and Ricordo J. Padilla, "Bisphosphonate-Related Osteonecrosis of the Jaws: A Report of Three Cases Demonstrating Variability in Outcomes and Morbidity," *Journal of the American Dental Association* 138(5):602–609, 2007.

Beatrice J. Edwards, MD, Mrinal Gounder, MD, June M. McKoy, MD, Ian Boyd, MD, et al., "Pharmacovigilance and Reporting Oversight in U.S. FDA Fast-Track Process: Bisphosphonates and Osteonecrosis of the Jaw," *The Lancet Oncology* 9(12):1166–72, 2008.

"Bone Health/Ostopenia," Dr. Susan Love Research Foundation, www.dslrf.org.

Dennis M. Black, Steven R. Cummings,

MD, David B. Karpf, MD, Jane A. Cauley, et al., "Randomised Trial of Effect of Alendronate on Risk of Fracture in Women with Existing Vertebral Fractures," *Lancet* 348(9041):1535–41, 1996.

Bone Health and Osteoporosis: A Report of the Surgeon General. Rockville, Maryland: U.S. Department of Health and Human Services, Public Health Service, Office of the Surgeon General, 2004.

Mary E. Tinetti, MD, Marki Speechley, and Sandra F. Ginter, "Risk Factors for Falls Among Elderly Persons Living in the Community," *New England Journal of Medicine* 319(1):701–707, 1988.

Susan Brink, "Treat? Or Wait? Fight Bone Loss Was a Mantra in the '90s. But Osteoporosis Knowledge Has Evolved. Sometimes, It's Better to Delay Drug Therapy," *Los Angeles Times,* September 22, 2008, p. F1.

Deborah Marshall, Olof Johnell, M.D, Hans Wedel, MD, "Meta-Analysis of How Well Measures of Bone Mineral Density Predict Occurrence of Osteoporotic Fractures," *BMJ* 312(7041):1254–1259, 1996.

Does Dad Really Have Alzheimer's?: A Look at Drug-Induced Dementia

Pekka K. Mölsä, MD, Reijo J. Marttila, MD, Urpo K. Rinne, MD, "Survival and Cause of Death in Alzheimer's Disease and Multi-Infarct Dementia," *Acta Neurologica Scandinavica* 74(2):103–107, 1986.

John Fauber, "Doubts Raised Over Drugs for Cholesterol; Side Effects Have Included Lost Memory in Some Patients," *Milwaukee Journal Sentinel,* March 28, 2004, p. 1A.

Duane Graveline, MD, *Lipitor, Thief of Memory: Statin Drugs and the Misguided War on Cholesterol.* Duane Gravelin, 2006.

Beatrice Alexander Golomb, MD, Michael H. Criqui, MD, Halbert White, and Joel E. Dimsdale, MD, "Conceptual Foundations of the UCSD [University of California, San Diego] Statin Study: A Randomized Controlled Trial Assessing the Impact of Statins on Cognition, Behavior, and Biochemistry," *Archives of Internal Medicine* 164:153–162, 2004.

Sharyl Attkisson, "Research Indicates Cholesterol-Lowering Statins Such as Lipitor May Cause Cognitive Dysfunctions in Some Patients," *CBS Evening News,* May 24, 2004.

Matthew F. Muldoon, MD, Christopher M. Ryan, Susan M. Sereika, Janine D. Flory, and Stephen B. Manuck, "Randomized Trial of the Effects of Simvastatin on Cognitive Functioning in Hypercholesterolemic Adults," *American Journal of Medicine* 117(11):823–829, 2004.

Matthew F. Muldoon, MD, Steven D. Barger, Christopher M. Ryan, Janine D. Flory, et al., "Effects of Lovastatin on Cognitive Function and Psychological Well-Being," *American Journal of Medicine* 108(7):538–546, 2000.

"Drugs That May Cause Psychiatric Symptoms," *Medical Letter on Drugs and Therapeutics* 44:59–62, 2002.

Anna Thalacker-Mercer, Melissa Baker, Chris Calderon, and Marcas Bamman, "Simvastatin Reduces Human Primary Satellite Cell Proliferation in Culture," presented at a conference of the American Physiological Society, September 24–27, 2008, Hilton Head, South Carolina.

Taking Charge: A Step-by-Step Guide to Controlling Your Medications (Rather than Letting Them Control You)

Irving Kirsch, Brett J. Deacon, Tania B. Huedo-Medina, Alan Scoboria, Thomas J. Moore, Blair T. Johnson, "Initial Severity and Antidepressant Benefits: A Meta-Analysis of Data Submitted to the Food and Drug Administration," *PLoS Medicine* 5(2):e45, 2008.

Debra Fulghum Bruce, "Facts About Antidepressants: A New Study Says Some Antidepressants Are Mostly Ineffective, But Many Previous Studies Show the Opposite," WebMD.com, February 28, 2008.

ACKNOWLEDGMENTS

"The success of a man," my dad always used to say as I was growing up, "is measured not by what he takes out of this world but by what he puts into it." In so many ways, I have my family to thank for instilling in me the desire and drive to help others. The love of my mom and dad, Mary Eleanor and Armon, Sr., has followed me and my two brothers, Charles and John, throughout our lives. Charles married Gloria, John married Sally, and I married June, with all of us celebrating fifty-plus years of marriage. My sons, Armon III and Camp, have brought their wives, Rebecca and Julie, into the family, giving us seven beautiful grandchildren: twins Elizabeth and Lindsey, Emily, Drake, Madison, and twins Grant and Alex. I tell everyone that if I had known that grandchildren were going to be so much fun, I would have had them first. With so much love around me I've had no choice but to always do my best and to always remember to put something into the world by helping others.

I've also been blessed to have many friends who have been positive influences on my life and career in pharmacy. I've known Terry Wynne, my lifelong best friend, since I was three years old. In addition to being college roommates (I was in pharmacy school and he was in optometry school), we served alongside each other in the Army and each played the role of best man in the other's wedding. Terry and I have shared so much that he's the best sounding board and confidant one could possibly hope to have. I also owe a lot to Frank Lindsey, who many years ago gave up his career as a banker to come work with me; he's the one who always keeps my wagon out of the ditch. Then there are some valued professional colleagues who are among the best pharmacists anywhere: Charles Feucht, of Eunice, Louisiana, and Peter Perrin, of Torrance, California, both of whom maintain practices similar to mine; Charlie Rinn, my sidekick in Columbus, Georgia, who not only gives me the benefit of his wisdom on pharmacy matters but who, with my brother Charles, has joined me in Miata rallies all over the country; Tom Clark, the executive director of the Commission for Certification in Geriatric Pharmacy, with whom I'm in contact almost constantly; Harlan Martin, of Clark, New Jersey, and Steve Feldman, of Boston Massachusetts, with whom I've worked closely for more than thirty years to introduce improvements in policies and procedures for older patients. I also owe much to the late Joseph LaRocca, the professor in pharmacy school who turned me on to medicinal chemistry — the science that's at the heart of pharmacology. And I want to acknowledge three pharmacists who helped me to change many laws and regulations that have improved the lives of millions of older Americans: Sam Kidder, who for many years was the chief of long-term care for the Health Care Financing Administration, and Stonewall King and the late Don Baker, who worked for HCFA's southern district office in Athens, Georgia.

I have many longtime colleagues to thank as well, chief among them the professional staff members of the consulting firm I founded: Dot Wynn, Shirley Glover, Jackie Brooks, and Patsy Smart, all registered nurses; Judith Longfellow, an occupational therapist; and the late Jody Thomas and his son, Steven Thomas, the computer pro-

451

grammers who developed our health-care records systems.

I have many physicians to thank, too. When I started out in geriatric care at Westbury Medical Home in Jackson, Georgia, I met the late R.V. Brandon, MD, the facility's medical director, who was paralyzed from the neck down as a result of an automobile accident. Dr. Brandon was the most gifted and most compassionate geriatrician I've ever encountered. He took me under his wing to teach me geriatrics, and I'll always be grateful for the twenty-plus years we worked together. Several other doctors that I worked closely with in the beginning of my career — including Tom Hunt, MD, the late J. Denny Hall, MD, and Tom Lipscomb, MD, all of Griffin, Georgia — also were wonderful teachers. Later in my career, doctors like Morris Davis, MD, of Tifton, Georgia, with whom I worked for thirty-plus years, helped make my experiences in nursing homes so educational and rewarding.

When I started the next chapter of my career with an outpatient practice in geriatric pharmacotherapy, two doctors in Griffin — James Gore, MD, and George Capo, D.O. — opened their doors to patients who needed help but were refused it by their previous doctors. Together we've watched many, many patients enjoy later years of their lives that had looked lost to them. Drs. Gore and Capo are truly life-savers.

In any long-term care facility, strong leadership is essential for the delivery of good patient care. Many in the Westbury family are strong leaders who oversee care that is second to none in the United States. Patsy Hightower Arline started as a dishwasher and as a single mother worked nights to become a certified nursing assistant, then a licensed practical nurse, and then a registered nurse — while putting her children through college. Now, as a licensed nursing home administrator, she sees to it that Westbury provides the kind of care that any of us would hope for if we had to go to a nursing home. Other pioneers in nursing home administration with whom I've been fortunate to work — among them Charles Templeton, Olitta Baggett, Bobby Tiner, Myrtle Vickers, Clark Peek, and Jimmy Pritchett — helped to make long-term care in Georgia light years ahead of that in many other states.

I often think that it took little pieces of all these wonderful people to make one Armon Neel, Jr., so my gratitude is enduring and heartfelt.

Finally, I wish to thank the many thousands of patients over the years who have trusted me to help them, even in cases where my advice ran counter to what they'd been told by other medical professionals. You've read some of their stories in this book, and I feel that they are really part of my family, too.

Armon B. Neel, Jr.
Griffin, Georgia
March 2012

We have many people to thank for helping to make this book a reality. Our collaboration is an outgrowth of a story for the *AARP Bulletin* ("The Pharmacist Who Says No to Drugs") that was published in September 2004. We met that summer, journalist and pharmacist, and in the years that followed became friends and then coauthors. Although we live seven hundred or so miles apart, it often seems to us that we're pretty much like next-door neighbors. We've shared a lot these past eight years, above all the drive to get an important message — the message that's at the core of this book — to a much larger audience.

Many people have helped along the way. Back in 2004, Bob Wilson, who was then the editor of the *AARP Bulletin,* encouraged me to write the story that became "The Pharmacist Who Says No to Drugs" and shepherded it into print; I'll always be mindful of how he started me on this journey. More recently, many of my other colleagues at AARP have helped — sometimes in ways they don't even appreciate — to keep me thinking, reporting, and writing about these issues, including: Kim Keister, a gifted editor who always knows just the right way to put the reader first; Teo Furtado, who originally hatched the idea for the "Ask the Pharmacist" column that we write for the AARP website and whose judgment about health-care stories is pitch-perfect; and Betsy Carpenter and Melissa Stanton, whose deft hands as editors have invariably improved our columns and other articles.

Armon and I are lucky to have had Gail Ross, a downright phenomenal literary agent (and lawyer), with us every step of the way. She believed in the book, and in us, from the beginning. We also are grateful to Howard Yoon, Gail's partner in the Ross Yoon literary agency, and to Anna Sproul, an editor there, for helping us to shape — and immeasurably improve — our original proposal for the book.

That proposal ultimately led to our first

meeting with Sarah Durand, the senior editor of Atria Books, and I remember Armon and I looking at each other as we emerged feeling as if we had found the perfect editor and the perfect home for our book. From the get-go, Sarah understood exactly what we wanted to do, and we feel extraordinarily fortunate to have had her as our editor. We also owe thanks to a number of other people at Atria Books, including Judith Curr, Alexandra Arnold, Ariele Fredman, Nancy Inglis, and Elisa Rivlin.

I've been blessed with the greatest friends anyone could ask for, and I want to thank a very special few who helped in ways big and small — mostly big — to keep me level-headed and in good spirits over the two-plus years that went into writing this book: Sergio Angeli, Blair Austin, Jane Cho, Alan Green, Joyce Knight, Nick Kotz, Sandy Kubler, Barbara Schecter, Kirk Victor, and Tom Wolff. I hope that I will be able to better repay all of you, now that I have a little more time on my hands.

Finally, I want to thank my beautiful family — Tom, Lucy, Bailey, and Cara — for all the happiness and fulfillment they've brought my way. I wouldn't have made it here without them.

Bill Hogan
Washington, D.C.
March 2012

INDEX

A

absorption, 66
acebutolol (Sectral), 293
ACE inhibitors, 69, 172–74, 186–87, 257
acetaminophen (Tylenol)
    diphenhydramine and, 278
    drug-drug interactions and, 71
    effectiveness of, 199, 204, 210
    liver damage and, 84
    side effects of, 165
acetylcholine, 69–70, 327, 343–44
acid reflux, 140, 216–17, 221–22, 234–39
    See also gastroesophageal reflux disease
        (GERD)
Adcal, 224
additive interactions, 70
adenocarcinoma, 228–29
ADME (absorption, distribution,
        metabolism, and excretion), 66–69
adverse effects of drugs
    ACE inhibitors and, 172–74

459

body chemistry and, 56, 60–69, 87
bone-renewal process and, 301–2
effects of, 56–57, 64, 75–77, 99, 283
NSAIDs and, 193, 194, 199–200, 210–11
pharmacodynamics and, 69–77
See also older people
Albafort, 224
albumin, 67–68, 195
albuterol inhalers, 340
alcohol use, 200, 273
aldrenate (Fosamax), 301, 307, 311, 315
allergy medicines, 278–79
allopurinol (Zyloprim), 258
alpha-adrenergic agonists, 183, 184
alpha-blockers, 168–69, 180, 186, 278, 339
alprazolam (Xanax), 117
Alzheimer, Alois, 325
Alzheimer's disease
  anticonvulsants and, 285
  antipsychotic drugs and, 113
  diagnosis of, 326, 328, 333, 339–46
  drug-induced symptoms, 327–28, 341,
    343, 345–46
  fears of, 325
  medications for treating, 342
  statins and, 251
  See also dementia
American Academy of Orthopaedic
    Surgeons Panel on Falls Prevention,
    291

BPH (benign prostatic hyperplasia)
  anticholinergic drugs and, 110
  clonidine and, 136
  doxazosin and, 145
  tamsulosin and, 84, 262, 278–79
British Geriatrics Society, 291
bromocriptine (Parlodel), 290
brompheniramine (Dimetane), 287–88
BRONJ (bisphosphonate-related
    osteonecrosis of the jaw), 312
bupropion (Wellbutrin), 120, 287
buttermilk, 235, 238

C
Cacit, 224
caffeine, side effects of, 165
Calcichew, 224
calcium carbonate supplements, 224, 317
calcium channel blockers, 171–72, 184,
    185, 196, 258
calcium citrate supplements, 317
Caltrate, 224
capillary fragility, 199
captopril (Capoten), 172
carbamazepine (Tegretol), 286
carbidopa-levodopa (Sinemet), 290
cardiac output, age-related changes in, 64
cardiovascular disease
  cholesterol and, 244, 246, 253–54,
    266–67

cholesterol
  alternatives for controlling, 272
  cardiovascular disease and, 244, 246,
    253–54, 266–67
  HDL cholesterol, 244–45, 259, 273
  LDL cholesterol, 241, 243–44, 259, 272
cholinergic properties, 71
chronic obstructive pulmonary disease
    (COPD), 125
cimetidine (Tagamet), 133–35, 213–14,
    224, 354
ciprofibrate (Modalim), 249
ciproflaxocin (Ciloxan, Cipro), 285
circadian rhythm, 237
citalopram (Celexa), 224, 287
clarithromycin (Biaxin), 224
clemastine (Tavist, Tavist-1), 288
clinical drug trials, 105, 187, 206
clonazepam (Klonopin), 286
clonidine (Catapres), 81, 136
clopidogrel (Plavix), 80, 83, 222, 224
clorazepate (Tranxene), 117, 299
Clostridium difficile diarrhea
  calcium carbonate supplements and, 317
  pantoprazole and, 48
  proton pump inhibitors and, 83, 216,
    229–30
clozapine (Clozaril), 292
Cochrane Collaboration, 247, 271

Cochrane Hypertension Review Group,
176
Cockcroft-Gault equation, 62
cognitive impairment
anesthesia and, 115, 328, 339, 349
chlordiazepoxide and, 335, 348–49
drug-induced, 327–28, 345–57
statins and, 250–51, 327, 328–32, 340,
350
thyroid gland and, 338
See also Alzheimer's disease; dementia
colchicine (Colcrys), 257, 258
Commission for Certification of Geriatric
Pharmacy, 375
compactin, 271
compliance, 167
congestive heart failure, 69
consultant pharmacists
drug therapy management and, 375,
388–90, 393, 395–96
Medicare and Medicaid programs and,
381–88
physicians and, 96–97, 103–4, 105, 135,
143, 203, 209, 382–3, 389–90,
397–98, 401–3
polypharmacy and, 86–87
tools for finding, 411
corticosteroid use
bone loss and, 303
cognitive impairment and, 353

dementia *(Cont.)*
  drug-induced dementia, 327–28, 333,
    339–40, 341, 343, 345–46
  palliative processes for, 334
  statins and, 251
  See also Alzheimer's disease
depression
  beta-blockers and, 170, 296, 348
  chlorzoxazone and, 133
  hypertension drugs and, 188
  mobility and, 199
  reserpine and, 157
  statins and, 251
  vitamin B12 deficiency and, 232
  See also antidepressants
desiccated thyroid (Armour Thyroid),
    138–39
desipramine (Norpramin), 287
dexamethasone (Decadron, Hexadrol,
    Mymethasone), 293
dexchlorpheniramine (Polaramine), 110
dextromethorphan (Delsym), 288
diabetes
  alpha-adrenergic agonists and, 184
  beta-blockers and, 171, 178, 181, 182,
    186
  drug-drug interactions and, 208
  drugs for treatment of, 53, 131–32, 186
  effect on kidney function, 69, 182
  hypoglycemia and, 131, 132, 280, 297

E

Eli Lilly and Company, 115
enalapril (Vasotec), 173, 288
enoxacin (Penetrex), 285
epilepsy, 115, 116
epoetin alfa (Procrit), 185
ergoloid mesylates (Hydergine), 146
escitalopram (Lexapro), 224, 287
esomeprazole (Nexium), 214, 240, 304
esophageal cancer, 229, 308
estazolam (ProSom), 117
estrogens (Premarin, Climara, Cenestin)
  Beers criteria, 119–22
  estrogen replacement therapy, 313
ethacrynic acid (Edecrin), 147
ethchlorvynol (Placidyl), 299
etodolac (Lodine), 296
excretion, 69, 76
exercise, 273, 282, 318

F

falls
  alpha-blockers and, 169
  benzodiazepines and, 117, 283, 299, 319
  causes of, 277, 284–99
  clonidine and, 135–37
  diphenhydramine and, 278
  dipyridamole, 141–42
  doxazosin and, 145
  drug-drug interactions and, 276–77, 291

G

Green, Lee A., 248
GR# (granulocyte count), 83
guanfacine (Intuniv), 169

H
H2 blockers
  acid reflux and, 140, 236
  Beers criteria and, 133–35
  cognitive impairment and, 354–55
  ferrous sulfate and, 148
  gastrointestinal disorders and, 157, 214
  proton pump inhibitors and, 224
haloperidol (Haldol), 111, 292, 335, 355
Hb (hemoglobin count), 83
HDL cholesterol, 244–45, 259, 273
Health Care Financing Administration, 103
health care system
  conflicts of interest and, 383, 385–86
  cost of diagnostic procedures, 378, 390
  cost of prescription drugs, 101, 381–82,
    385, 390, 393–96
  infant morality and, 379
  life expectancy and, 379–80
  nursing homes and, 381–88
  preventive care and, 379, 380
  quick-fix response promoted by, 51
  survey of primary care physicians,
    380–81
Heart UK, 242
hemogloblin (Hgb), 185

479

Lantus, 185
LDL cholesterol, 241, 243–44, 259, 272
L-dopa, 290
lean muscle mass/body fat ratio, 65, 66–67,
    136
Lemmon, Robert, 243, 246
levobunolol (Betagan), 297
levodopa (Larodopa), 290
levofloxacin (Levaquin), 285
levothyroxine (Levoxyl, Synthroid), 138,
    338
lisinopril (Prinivil, Zestril), 172–73
liver
  acetaminophen and, 84
  age-related changes in, 59, 64, 68, 283,
      328
  amiodarone and, 124
  antidepressants and, 286
  benzodiazepines and, 117, 298–99, 349
  beta-blockers and, 178, 292–93
  calcium channel blockers and, 172
  chlorzoxazone and, 132
  cholesterol and, 244
  cimetidine and, 134
  CYP2D6, 178, 286, 292–93
  CYP3A4, 172, 253
  fluoxetine and, 148
  functions of, 59
  H2 blockers and, 214
  hypertension drugs and, 187

melatonin supplements, 237–38
meloxicam (Mobic), 122, 140, 208
meperidine (Demerol), 150–51, 349
meprobamate (Miltown, Equanil), 129,
    151, 299
Merck, 206, 271, 315
Merck Manuals, 97
mesoridazine (Serentil), 111
metabolism
  accumulation of drugs and, 117, 298–99,
      328
  metabolic rate changes, 57
  as pharmacokinetic process, 65–66, 68,
      76, 89–90, 91
  proton pump inhibitors and, 223
  statins and, 253
metaxalone (Skelaxin), 151–52
metformin (Glucophage), 53, 182, 357
methocarbamol (Robaxin), 152, 295
methotrexate (Rheumatrex, Trexall), 224
methyldopa (Aldomet), 152
methylphenidate (Ritalin), 108, 264
methylprednisone (Medrol), 293
methyprylon (Noludar), 299
metipranolol (Optipranolol), 297
metoprolol (Betaloc, Toprol, Toprol XL,
    Lopressor)
  as beta-blocker, 80, 81, 170
  cognitive impairment and, 348
  falls and, 289, 292

P

palliative care, for older people, 97
pantoprazole (Protonix)
  bone loss and, 304–5
  Clostridium difficile and, 48
  as proton pump inhibitor, 80, 209, 214
parkinsonism, 113, 156, 289, 291
Parkinson's disease, 289–90
paroxetine (Paxil), 287, 368
penbutolol (Levatol), 170, 293
penicillins, 225
pentazocine (Talwin), 155
pentoxifylline (Trental), 79, 83
perphenazine-amitriptyline (Triavil), 112,
    155–56
personal medication dossier, 361–63, 375
Pfizer, 206, 211, 327
pharmaceutical manufacturers
  bisphosphonates and, 301
  cost of drugs and, 381
  information provided by, 101, 170, 188,
    242, 246
  marketing campaigns of, 205–6, 210–11
pharmacists
  geriatric pharmacists, 375, 399, 405, 411
  instructions on prescription drugs,
    371–74
  retail pharmacists, 383
  See also consultant pharmacists
pharmacodynamics, 69–77, 105

hypomagnesemia risk and, 227–28
pneumonia and, 216, 231
propantheline and, 157
rebound acid hypersecretion, 218, 220
as short-term therapeutic intervention,
218, 222
side effects of, 47–48, 83, 140, 215–16,
223–32, 238–39, 355
ulcers and, 230, 232, 233
vitamin B12 deficiency and, 216, 231–32
psychiatrists, 100
Public Citizen's Health Research Group,
412–13
pulmonary fibrosis, 124, 153, 155
pulmonary function, 64

Q
quazepam (Doral, Dormalin), 117
quetiapine (Seroquel), 112, 356
quinapril (Accupril), 173
quinidine (Quinidex), 144

R
rabeprazole (Aciphex), 214
ramipril (Altace, Tritace), 173, 289
ranitidine (Zantac), 214, 224, 236
Raynaud's disease, 54, 150, 171, 181
RBC (red blood cell count), 83
rebound acid hypersecretion, 218, 220
rebound acidosis, 317

rebound effect, 309

Reckless, John, 242

reserpine (Serpalan, Serpasil), 157

restless leg syndrome (RLS), 46, 254, 256, 289, 350

retail pharmacists, 383

rhabdomyolysis, 249, 258, 260

risedronate (Actone), 301

risperidone (Risperdal), 112, 292, 355–56, 387

rivaroxaban (Xarelto), 202

Roche Group, 302

rofecoxib (Vioxx), 201, 205–6

ropinirole (Requip), 255, 290

rosuvastatin (Crestor), 203–4, 241, 350

S

Schedule II controlled substances, 108

Schedule IV controlled substances, 129

schizophrenia, 112

scopolamine (Scopace), 213

sedative hypnotics, 102, 353

selective serotonin reuptake inhibitors (SSRIs), 149, 286

selegiline (Eldepryl), 290

self-assessment quiz, 405–10

senile tremors, 116

sensory changes, 57

sertraline (Zoloft), 287

simvastatin (Zocor, Vytorin), 241, 250, 350

U

ulcers, proton pump inhibitors and, 230, 232, 233

V

valdecoxib (Bextra), 80, 201–2, 206
valproate (Epilim), 286
valsartan (Diovan), 175
vasodilators, 181, 183, 184
venlafaxine (Effexor XR), 81, 121, 368
verapamil (Anpec, Isoptin), 289
vitamin B12 deficiency, 216, 231–32, 274
vitamin-B-complex therapy, 245, 258, 274
vitamin D supplements, 282–83, 317, 318

W

Wallace, John, 232
warfarin (Coumadin), 67, 201–2, 208, 225
water-soluble medications, 67
WBC (white blood cell count), 83
West, Tony, 387–88
West of Scotland Coronary Prevention Study (WOSCOPS), 265–70
white-coat hypertension, 163
Wolfe, Sidney M., 220
World Health Organization, 160
WorstPills.org, 412

Y

yogurt, 236, 238

Z

The employees of Thorndike Press hope you have enjoyed this Large Print book. All our Thorndike, Wheeler, and Kennebec Large Print titles are designed for easy reading, and all our books are made to last. Other Thorndike Press Large Print books are available at your library, through selected bookstores, or directly from us.

For information about titles, please call:
 (800) 223-1244

or visit our Web site at:
 http://gale.cengage.com/thorndike

To share your comments, please write:
 Publisher
 Thorndike Press
 10 Water St., Suite 310
 Waterville, ME 04901